Get Strong, Lean, and Serene with

EASY WEIGHT LOSS YOGA 2
INTERMEDIATE

Poses and Sequences for Stamina, Balance, Relaxation, and Fat-Burning

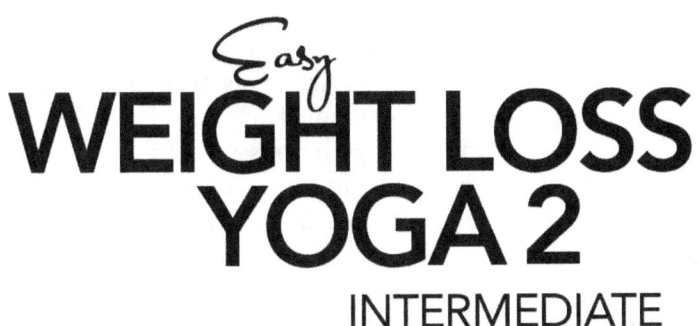

Easy WEIGHT LOSS YOGA 2

INTERMEDIATE

PATRICIA BACALL

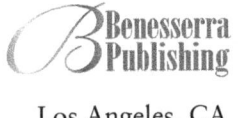

Benesserra Publishing

Los Angeles, CA

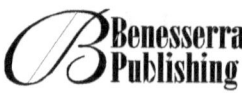

1827 Barry Ave., Los Angeles, CA 90025, 800-931-7007
First Edition
Paperback ISBN: 978-1-4961423-1-3
Ebook ISBN: 978-0-9884917-9-3

DISCLAIMER

The purpose of this book is that of education and entertainment, and it is not intended as a substitute for the advice and guidance of a qualified yoga teacher or the medical advice of physicians. The reader should regularly consult a physician in matters relating to his/her health, particularly with respect to any symptoms that may require diagnosis or medical attention.

Always consult your physician before beginning any exercise program. This general information is not intended to diagnose any medical condition or to replace your healthcare professional. Consult with your healthcare professional to design an appropriate exercise prescription. Always work within your own range of limits and abilities. If you have any medical concerns, talk with your doctor before practicing yoga. If you experience any pain or difficulty with these exercises, stop and consult your healthcare provider. Common sense and caution should be used when embarking on any physically demanding endeavor.

Contents

INTRODUCTION

What You'll Gain from Reading This Book (and What You'll Lose!)

For readers of Easy Weight Loss Yoga: 12 Best Poses to Get Lean, Strong, and Calm, this book is the next step in normalizing your weight without having to resort to the dreary up-and-down Ferris wheel of weight loss and gain, or the sad merry-go-round of food restriction and dieting. For readers who are new to Easy Weight Loss Yoga, the book will provide not only the best poses for tuning up your metabolism to become a lean, mean, fat-burning machine, but also the poses combined in the best, most effective sequences for building stamina, working on balance, fat burning, and relaxation. While you can also include poses for each in one yoga session, I find it worthwhile to be able to focus on one capability per session and have slightly shorter sessions. While there are poses that you'll want to include in every yoga session, I think it's helpful to work on becoming a specialist rather than a generalist. By specializing, you will know enough about each pose and what it does to be able to combine them on your own, according to what you feel you need on any given day.

As you progress in your Easy Yoga practice, you'll begin to notice an increase in your energy, breathing, and flexibility of both body and mind. In all my books, I talk about not continuously monitoring your weight to see if the scale has moved. Instead, move forward into your new yoga lifestyle with enthusiasm and confidently assume that the desired changes will come simply as a result of your intention and the changes you're making. Just as you wouldn't continuously uproot a seedling to see if it's growing, don't continually jump on the scale to weigh in. Be patient and kind to yourself and the extra weight will begin to just drop away. As you get more into the yoga lifestyle, you'll be eliminating the fears and concerns about your body and weight that you formerly obsessed over. You're planting the seeds of your future best self. Yoga will give you freedom to be that best self and grow continuously.

Yoga is best practiced with the intention to engage in self-exploration with a certain degree of curiosity about what each session will reveal and not to necessarily get "better" at it. Of course you want to achieve your goals of feeling good and losing weight, but if you approach the mat with the intention to do as well as you can in this moment, the results will simply start occurring. You'll reap the rewards without the stress of self-judgment. The gentle approach of practicing to achieve better overall health will serve you better than focusing on the specific goal of weight loss; it's a lifestyle change you are seeking.

WHAT YOGA CAN DO FOR YOU: BENEFITS OF THE YOGIC LIFESTYLE TO ALL ASPECTS OF YOUR LIFE

Yoga is not goal-oriented, dogmatic, a religion, or anything that needs to be adhered to rigidly—it's simply a way of living where the aim is "a healthy mind in a healthy body." Yoga does not interfere with or undermine any religious beliefs or values that you already hold.

Understanding that we are physical, mental, and spiritual beings, yoga helps promote a balanced development of all three. Yoga becomes a lifestyle choice as the benefits accrue. As you begin to experience more serenity and wellness, you'll naturally want to experience more happiness and bliss. We humans are just built that way. We're pleasure seekers. Fortunately, yoga offers healthy and beneficial pleasure-seeking behavior, drawing you along a path to greater serenity and enjoyment. (And in my humble opinion, it's a far cry from the unconscious stupor many people like to think is pleasure.)

Other forms of physical exercise, like aerobics, promote physical well-being but have little to do with the development of the emotional and/or spiritual body. Yoga develops you in a holistic way. You can't do just the callisthenic part of yoga without including conscious breathing, nor can you hold postures without noticing how it feels in your body. One part of your yoga practice flows into the next and all work together to heighten your awareness of yourself. If you allow it, you'll begin to notice that you react the same way in life as you do on the mat, and you can use that information to make changes for the better.

Yoga can literally change the chemistry of the body and therefore recharge it with life-force energy, which in turn:

- facilitates attainment of harmony and equilibrium;

- promotes self-healing;

- removes negative blocks from the mind and toxins from the body;

- enhances personal power;

- increases self-awareness;

- helps in attention focus and concentration; and

- reduces stress and tension in the physical body by activating the parasympathetic nervous system.

By practicing yoga, you will feel rejuvenated and energized, and, depending on the structure and sequencing of the postures you choose, your practice can focus on relaxation, balance, building strength and stamina, or increasing flexibility.

CHAPTER 1

Yoga — The Marriage of Movement and Breath

YOGA IS BREATHING WITH POSTURES, NOT THE OTHER WAY AROUND

First, a few words about breathing and its importance. As you may know, the word yoga means "union." It is well known and generally assumed that it is a union between body, mind, and soul; but somewhat less well known is that it's also a union between movement and breathing. During our sequences, we attempt to create a marriage between the movements and the breath, to create one unbroken and even flow to the poses, so that the breath is either an "inflow" or an "outflow" with each movement.

Every moment of your yoga practice is filled with breathing, except for the final resting pose, or Corpse Pose, where you allow your breathing to simply become very quiet and soft. The yogic term for specialized breathing is pranayama, which literally means "to extend the vital life force." It is an incredibly rich practice made up of many breathing techniques that vary in complexity from ones simple enough for a child to do to those appropriate for only advanced practitioners.

In my many years of teaching yoga and breathwork, I've seen simple breathing practices reduce stress and anxiety; promote more restful sleep; ease pain; increase attention and focus; and, on a more subtle level, help people connect to a calm, quiet place within so they can experience greater clarity and well-being on every level. As a Vivation breathwork professional, I've seen amazing inner healing occur, as a result of the process, with conditions such as post-traumatic stress disorder, compulsive behavior, and emotional healing from wounds so deep that the person couldn't even begin to talk about the pain. Breathing is an important component in any healing process and deserves heightened attention during your yoga session.

The author of the Yoga Sutras, Patanjali, describes pranayama as a process by which you can break your unconscious breathing pattern and make the breath easy and smooth. Most people's unconscious breathing patterns are anything but easy and smooth; they tend to be tense, shallow, and erratic. When we are afraid or hear bad news, we often gasp—inhaling and then holding the breath. These breathing patterns can activate the sympathetic nervous system, often referred to as the "fight or flight response." To develop any new breathing pattern, first we must be aware of the breath.

One of the primary reasons that yogic breathing techniques suggest a long, smooth inhale and exhale is because, when practiced correctly, it can support the parasympathetic nervous system and activate what is commonly known as the "relaxation response," reducing stress and its effects on your body and mind. As a result, your resilience in the face of challenge or adversity increases and your mind becomes more focused and still.

QUIETING THE MIND

One of the other very important aspects in utilizing the breath is that breathing is a path to help you reach the state of yoga (union), or focused concentration. But this focused concentration is not the end goal. The more important result of reaching this state of attention is that you experience clearer perception and a greater connection with your true self. When you're connected with your true self, it becomes easier to see what is not your true self—your mind, body, thoughts, feelings, job, and essentially all the changing circumstances around you. This discernment allows you to act from a place of centeredness, and when you do that, you experience less suffering.

Breathing is an important tool to get you to this state of more focused concentration, leading you to clearer perception, a greater connection with the self, and ultimately a happier life. As Patanjali writes, "As a result of pranayama, the covering that blocks our own inner light is reduced." In other words, through the practice of pranayama, you can reduce all of the mental noise—the agitation, distractions, and self-doubt—that prevents you from connecting with your own inner light, your true self. In this way, pranayama can have a profound effect on your life.[1]

During the yoga postures and sequences, all breathing is done through the nose, which warms the lungs on the inhale and retains the warmth in the body on the exhale. The breath is drawn deep into the lungs, so you can feel your ribs expand with each breath. You have to be conscious of the breath because "deep and continuous" is not our natural way to breathe. Finally, the breath is relaxed and not forced in any way. True, the breath has to be conscious and intentional, but that isn't the same as forced. If someone were listening to you without being able to see you, they would think that you were simply relaxing, doing deep breathing. In other words, no grunting, groaning, pursing the lips, blowing, holding the breath, gasping, moaning, et cetera. Imagine a sleeping baby's breathing and try to consciously imitate that throughout your entire yoga session. You don't need to breathe particularly slowly in yoga. If the pose demands more prana (more air or energy), just breathe faster in and out through your nose. Don't be afraid to back off from the intensity of the pose if it makes you too breathless or exhausted.

---

1   Kate Holcombe, *Yoga Journal, August 2012*

CHAPTER 2

An Overview of the History of Yoga

DEFINITIONS OF YOGA

Whether you get into yoga for physical exercise, weight loss, relaxation, or rehabilitation, it's worthwhile to know a little about the history of yoga and its lineage of esoteric thought. Yoga is not simply upward and downward dog poses, as many people think, and it can be confusing to the novice to see so many kinds of different yoga styles. Which one will be the right one for you? By knowing a bit about how yoga has evolved, you'll be able to see how the different schools developed and understand the differences.

Yoga is a multi-dimensional practice, and the distinction of each aspect is somewhat important to understand, based on what you want yoga to do for you.

The formal definitions of yoga are:

A Hindu theistic philosophy teaching the suppression of all activity of body, mind, and will, in order that the self may realize its distinction from them and attain liberation. (This is what we think of when we see pictures of monastic East Indians, clothed in only a loincloth.) In the West, some aspects of this definition are brought into the everyday practice of yoga by teachers in studios and health clubs. Normally,

9

however, the concept of withdrawal from the senses is not emphasized, and it is assumed that simply in the practice of yoga (as in the following definition) that yoga itself has the inherent power to bring about the desired evolution for the individual. Yoga is, of course, a valid path to liberation or enlightenment, but it is not for this purpose that most Westerners are drawn to practice yoga.

A system of physical postures, breathing techniques, and meditation, derived from yoga but often practiced independently, especially in Western cultures, to promote bodily or mental control and well-being. It is this second definition with which most yoga recruits are familiar, so just for a moment, let's delve into the history of yoga, so you can understand its origins and true capabilities.

You probably already have an idea of why you're drawn to yoga, but to give you an even richer feeling for what you already know, you should be aware of its roots and beginnings. As a dedicated yogi (which you are if you are reading this sequel to Easy Weight Loss Yoga), taking a look at the history of yoga will allow you to appreciate its rich tradition, as well as help you understand to what extent you would like to incorporate even more yoga philosophy into your life.

Although some say that yoga is "as old as civilization itself," there is no physical evidence to support this claim. Stone seals, which are the earliest archaeological evidence of yoga's existence, depict figures of yoga poses and place yoga's emergence at around 3000 B.C.[2]

However, scholars have reason to believe that yoga existed long before that and can trace its beginnings to Stone Age shamanism. Both shamanism and yoga have similar characteristics, specifically their efforts to improve the human condition. Also, they aim to heal community members, with the yogis and shamans acting as religious mediators. Although we think of yoga as focusing more on the self, it started out being community-oriented before it turned inward.[3]

The Vedic Period

The Vedic civilization is associated with the period of the origination of the Vedas, the earliest known spiritual texts. The Vedas are still influencing spiritual and philosophical belief today through their contribution to yoga. They are the sacred scriptures of Brahmanism, which are the basis of modern-day Hinduism. The Vedas are a collection of hymns that praise the divine power. They contain the oldest known yogic teachings, which are characterized by rituals and ceremonies that strive to surpass the limitations of the mind. This is important to note because it is the cessation of the perception of suffering, created in

---

2   *Shaynebance, abc-of-yoga.com*
3   *Wikipedia, Shamanism and Yoga, 2013*

the mind, that allows us to transcend our limitations and achieve happiness and serenity through our yoga practice.

During this time, the Vedic people relied on rishis, or dedicated Vedic yogis, to teach them how to live in divine harmony. Rishis were thought to be gifted with the ability to see the ultimate reality because of their intensive spiritual practice. The term rishi originates from the ancient pre-Hindu culture of the Indus-region earth-based cultures. A rishi is a sage of insight, one who practices self-cultivation as a yogi to attain a state of mental, emotional, and spiritual freedom called samadhi. Through concentration, he or she can attain realization of the independence of soul and body, and with continued effort attain realization of oneness with all.[4]

PRE-CLASSICAL PERIOD

The creation of the Upanishads (meaning "sitting near," with the intention of receiving esoteric teachings) marks the Pre-Classical Yoga period. The Upanishads are an amazing collection of writings from original oral transmissions, which have been described by famous yoga teacher Sri Aurobindo as "the supreme work of the Indian mind." The two hundred scriptures of the Upanishads describe the inner vision of reality resulting from devotion to a Supreme Intelligence, or

4   *Wikipedia, Rishis, Yoga, 2013*

Brahman. They explain three subjects: the ultimate reality (Brahman), the transcendental self (atman), and the relationship between the two.

It is here that we find all the fundamental teachings that are central to Hinduism—the concepts of karma (action), samsara (reincarnation), moksha (nirvana), the atman (soul), and the Brahman (the Absolute). They also set forth the prime Vedic doctrines of self-realization, yoga, and meditation. The Upanishads are summits of thought on mankind and the universe, designed to push human ideas to their very limit and beyond. They give us both spiritual vision and philosophical argument, stating that it is by strictly personal effort that one can reach the truth.[5]

Yoga shares some characteristics not only with Hinduism but also with Buddhism. Siddharta Gautama, the first Buddhist to study yoga, achieved enlightenment at the age of thirty-five. Then, during the sixth century B.C., Buddha started teaching Buddhism, which stresses the importance of meditation and the practice of physical postures. Later, around 500 B.C., the Bhagavad-Gita was created, and this is currently the oldest known yoga scripture. The central point to the Gita is that to be alive means to be active, and in order to avoid creating suffering in our lives and in others, our actions must be benign and must exceed our egos. (Ego can be defined as an individual's sense

---

5   *About.com/Hinduism*

of self, a person's self-esteem or self-importance, or the part of the mind that mediates between the conscious and the unconscious. The ego is responsible for reality testing and a sense of personal identity.)

British philosopher and mystic Paul Brunton explains, "One important reason why the great spiritual teachers have always enjoined upon their disciples the need of surrendering the ego, of giving up the self, is that when the mind is continually preoccupied with its own personal affairs, it sets up a narrow limitation upon its own possibilities. It cannot reach towards an impersonal truth, which is so different and so distant from the topics that it thinks about day after day, year after year. Only by breaking through its self-imposed pettiness can the human mind enter into the perception of the Infinite, of the divine soul that is its innermost being. No ordinary man really knows himself. He knows only his idea of himself. The two are not the same. If he wants to know his true self, he must first liberate himself from this false one, this imagined one, this idea."[6]

Just as the Upanishads further the Vedas, the Bhagavad-Gita builds on and incorporates the doctrines found in the Upanishads. In the Gita, three facets must be brought together in our lifestyle: Bhakti (loving devotion), Jnana (knowledge or contemplation), and

---

6   Paul Brunton, *Notebooks of Paul Brunton, Chapter 4: Detaching from The Ego,* *http://wisdomsgoldenrod.org/notebooks/8/4*

Karma (about selfless actions). The Gita then tried to unify Bhakti Yoga, Jnana Yoga, and Karma Yoga, and it is because of this that the Bhagavad-Gita has gained importance.

Classical Period

The Classical period is marked by another literary creation—the Yoga Sutras. Written by Patanjali around the second century, these were an attempt to define and standardize classical yoga. It is composed of sutras (from the Sanskrit word meaning "thread") that expound upon Raja Yoga and its underlying principles. Patanjali's Eightfold Path of Yoga (also called Eight Limbs of Classical Yoga) are:

1. Yama, social restraints or ethical values;
2. Niyama, personal observances of purity, tolerance, and study;
3. Asanas, or physical exercises;
4. Pranayama, breath control or regulation;
5. Pratyahara, or sense withdrawal in preparation for meditation;
6. Dharana, concentration;
7. Dhyana, meditation; and
8. Samadhi, ecstasy.

Patanjali believed that each individual is a composite of matter (prakriti) and spirit. He further that the two must be separated in order to cleanse the spirit—a stark contrast to Vedic and Pre-Classical Yoga, which signify the union of body and spirit.

Patanjali's concept was so dominant that, for some time, some yogis focused exclusively on meditation and neglected their asanas (yoga postures). It was only later that the belief of the body as a temple was rekindled and attention to the importance of the practice of asana was revived. (It is interesting to note that, at this time, yogis attempted to use yoga techniques to change the energetic composition of the body and make it immortal.)

Post-Classical Yoga

Post-Classical Yoga differs from the first three since its focus is more on the present. It no longer strives to liberate a person from reality but rather teaches one to accept it and live in the moment.

The yoga teachings that emerged in the period after Patanjali, which did not adopt his dualistic philosophy, can collectively be called Post-Classical Yoga. In contrast to other types of yoga, Post-Classical Yoga does not try to liberate a person from reality, but encourages attention on the present. The Post-Classical era saw an increase in literature and many branches of yoga, such as Tantra Yoga (out of which grew Siddha and Hatha Yoga, or body yoga). What was different, however, was the rejection of Patanjali's dualistic views.

Modern Yoga

Yoga was introduced in the West during the early nineteenth century. It was first studied as part of Eastern Philosophy and began as a movement for health and vegetarianism in the 1930s. Modern yoga is considered to have begun when Swami Vivekananda appeared at the Parliament of Religions in Chicago in 1893, a move that marked the beginning of yoga's migration into the West. As one of the chief yoga practitioners with a Western education, Vivekananda was pivotal in sharing the wisdom of yoga with an international audience. Handsome, charming, and articulate, he played on America's fascination with the exotic. His success rested on his unique ability to defuse the religious tensions that materialized when yoga met Christianity. Vivekananda was able to resolve these tensions by disassociating the practice of yoga from its popular conception of a practice primarily for Hindu men and instead associating it with health in general.[7][8]

By the 1960s, there was an influx of Indian teachers who expounded on yoga. One of them was Maharishi Mahesh, the yogi who popularized Transcendental Meditation. Another teacher was a prominent yoga guru, Swami Sivananda. Sivananda was a doctor in Malaysia who later opened yoga schools in America

7 Douglass, Laura. 2007. "The Yoga Tradition: How Did We Get Here? A History of Yoga in America, 1800-1970." *International Journal of Yoga Therapy.* 17: 35-42.

8 http://www.randomhistory.com/2009/01/27_yoga.html

and Europe. Sivananda wrote more than two hundred books on yoga and philosophy and had many disciples who furthered yoga. Some of these disciples included Swami Satchitananda, who introduced chanting and yoga to Woodstock (the Beatles' interest in yoga—particularly George Harrison and his wife's involvement—was partly responsible for popularizing it in the West[9]), Swami Sivananada Radha, who explored the connection between psychology and yoga, and Yogi Bhajan, who started teaching Kundalini Yoga in the 1970s.

The image of yoga as a discipline for greater health and vitality gradually led scholars to turn their attention to yoga's relationship to the body in the 1990s, and this has evolved into the current focus on its medical and psychological benefits. To this day, yoga continues to proliferate and spread its teachings, crossing the boundaries of culture and language in various forms. No one style of yoga is right for everyone, and you must find the type of yoga with which you resonate best. The simplest way to do this is to visit various studios and ask about the primary style of yoga they teach, then join a class and see if you like it.

9   Lennon, Cynthia. "The Beatles, the Maharishi, and Me." *TimesOnline. com. February 10, 2008. Accessed: November 11, 2008.*

CHAPTER 3

Your Yoga Practice

You don't need a fancy setup to begin practicing yoga. All you need is comfortable clothing (most yogis prefer tops that fit close to the body, so they don't slide up and cover your face in inverted poses such as Downward Facing Dog) and a yoga mat or sticky mat. Most people like to do yoga barefoot, but it is possible to wear socks, soft shoes, or footwear specially made for yoga (these include some kind of traction material on the bottom). Personally, I like the freedom of bare feet on a yoga mat, but you can experiment with various footwear if you don't like going barefoot. If you practice on a hard floor with socks, your feet may slip when in a pose such as Downward Facing Dog, thus the need for the mat. Keep your mat clean by wiping it down occasionally with a mild cleaner or diluted vinegar, and always fold it in half before you roll it up to keep the dirt of the floor off the surface on which you practice.

On a side note, some people consider their yoga mat a place of worship, therefore sacred, so it is good etiquette to avoid walking on other yogi's mats when in a yoga class, if possible. If you tend to drip sweat and your mat gets too slippery, try one of the moisture absorbing mat liners or a large towel on top of your yoga mat. A towel is always good to keep handy anyway, since you can use it as a prop to help you get into a pose, such as forward bend, if you're not flexible enough. Also, if you plan on taking a yoga class, try to avoid wearing perfume, as it bothers people with allergies. You can light candles and play any kind of meditative music you like if it helps you relax, as long as it isn't distracting and doesn't take your attention away from your practice.

GETTING STARTED

The best way to get started is to just make the decision to start where you're at, as if this is the first day of the rest of your life and you're open to experiencing anything. Adopt "Beginner's Mind"—an inviting, expectant awareness of curiosity and adventure. One of my favorite motivational sayings is, "Something is Better than Nothing," and I use it often, thinking, I'll just get started and do a little bit. If nothing else, I'll have done at least some yoga. Sometimes the hardest part of a yoga session is getting started—making the space for yourself to practice by turning the phone off and stopping the ceaseless "to-do's" that we all have.

Start your yoga session by bringing an intention into your consciousness of what you want to create in your session. It could be an intention to complete a certain sequence, master a specific posture, create a sense of well-being, relax, or even the thought of, I'm going to allow my subconscious to dictate this session and see what happens. Then, as Carlos Castenada's shaman, Don Juan, would say, "Stop the world." Meaning, become aware of your thoughts, be aware of your place in the present moment, become mindful of your body, your surroundings, your breath. In other words, check in with yourself and simply notice where you exist at this, the start of your yoga session. Start focusing your conscious awareness on your breathing, and once you start to settle in, then begin your postures. Don't treat your yoga session as simply just one more thing to do in your day of activities. Be present.

Decide on the postures you will do this session. Ease in with your feeling sense, being gentle with yourself. Don't fall into the trap of allowing your mind to dictate what the intensity of your session will be on a given day. The way we treat our bodies during yoga is a manifestation of how we feel about ourselves. Don't be unkind to your hamstring because it's tighter than you'd like it to be. Instead, grant your muscle compassion and breath, and it will begin to loosen up. There will be times when you won't practice for a week, and when you begin again, you may not be as strong or flexible. That's okay. Allow yourself to be exactly where you're at, and before you know it, your strength and flexibility will return. Only the internal dialogue of chastisement can keep you from enjoying your practice—nothing else. Simply start and be as kind to your body as you would be to a beloved child or pet. Extend the same gentleness and warmth, and your body will love you for it.

ON BEING "GOOD" AT YOGA

After a few weeks or months of practicing the poses, you will notice that some have gotten easy for you, some much more than others. We all have inherent strengths and weaknesses that the yoga poses will highlight, showing you what needs a little more attention. Spending time practicing your more challenging poses will be time well spent, giving you a feeling of accomplishment. But there are always new challenges in yoga, so learn to not rest on your laurels. Being "good" at yoga postures is something that doesn't exist. Remember, yoga is a practice that helps us to deeply explore ourselves while learning to quiet the mind. The "Yoga Olympics" doesn't exist. Allow yourself to grow with your practice, and just let go! You don't benefit by thinking of how good you are at any given moment in your yoga career. One never graduates, and there is always someone better than you at any pose. Yoga teaches you humility, because just as you begin to congratulate yourself on how well you're doing a posture, you fall over.

There's enough pressure everywhere to be good, to be perfect, to get it right—you don't need your yoga practice to be another competition. Always act as the impeccable warrior you are and do the best you can, but don't get cocky. Let go of any competitiveness, close your eyes, and flow. Some days will feel great, and some days will be difficult and you'll feel like stopping. Don't. Don't judge your practice, don't decide it's not working or that nothing is happening. Welcome yoga in and let the poses take you somewhere magnificent, just as they've done for thousands of people for thousands of years. You deserve to communicate deeply with your body, to strengthen yourself inside and out, and to change all that does not serve you.[10]

FINDING MOTIVATION

Even if you don't have time for sixty- or ninety-minute classes in your schedule, just twenty to thirty minutes a day of yoga practice will have a very significant effect on your health, weight, and well-being.

It's always good to challenge yourself to do the best you can at any time, but it's never to your benefit to push yourself past the point of discomfort and into pain. My motto has always been, "Live to practice another day." Injuries can be a tough way to learn the lesson of being gentle with yourself. Use common sense, err on the side of caution, and remember that doing yoga with awareness and without injuries will give you the strength and confidence to go further in your next session on the mat.

---

10 *Diana Scime-Sayegh, mindbodygreen.com, October 31, 2013*

Even a short sequence of postures will help anyone who adds it to his or her daily life. How can I be so sure of this? Well, SIBTN! (Something is Better than Nothing.) Because human beings didn't evolve to sit or lie down twenty-four hours a day, any movement is better than none. Our ancestors had to bend and lift and chop and jump and run and climb daily just to survive, and obesity was rare. Even if you are over-weight and need to start off very slowly with your practice, the benefits will accumulate.

The only way to lose weight and keep it off for the rest of your life is by changing your lifestyle and adopting a healthy one, which includes the joys and challenges of moving, breathing properly, continu-ously feeding yourself "alivening" foods, and learning to avoid the temptation of overindulging in "dead-ening" foods or toxic substances. By accepting the discipline, you'll improve your chances for living a longer, happier, healthier life. The yogic lifestyle will cause you to grow as a person mentally, physically, emotionally, and spiritually. This is the main reason to practice, not just to lose weight for vanity's sake, but to evolve as a fearless, fully actualized person who can be both self-reliant and sensitive, empathetic to others, strong, and in tune with the greater purpose of improving life on earth.

CHAPTER 4

Yoga and Weight Loss

Yoga is perfect for weight loss because it's more than just a physical workout; it will help you deal with stress in your life without resorting to food to energize or soothe yourself. Yoga tunes up your entire system and makes it function better. Your first goal for achieving lasting weight loss is to get as healthy as you can. Knowing what systems are affected will help you understand why this is necessary and ultimately achieve this most important goal.

There are different types of Asana (physical) yoga that can help with weight loss, such as Hatha, Ashtanga, Vinyasa Flow, and Power Yoga. Some types help with weight loss more than others because of the caloric expenditure involved, but your yoga practice for weight loss does not have to be extremely strenuous to work well for you. Gentle Hatha Yoga, and even seated Chair Yoga, will give many health benefits and can be helpful with weight loss because you are triggering the parasympathetic nervous system, which regulates breathing, digestion, and hormones.

Depending on the type of yoga you perform, calories burned during your workout can vary from 180 to 360 calories per hour. Power Yoga is often the common choice for weight loss because of its triple forces, including strength, flexibility, and cardio, but every kind of Hatha Yoga can be beneficial. In a typical sixty- to ninety-minute session, you will have touched almost all the muscles, ligaments, organs, glands, and bones of the body in some way. The deep breathing techniques used in coordination with the postures help flush out toxins and water weight. Yoga also boosts the lymphatic system and encourages it to perform better.

Weight loss is the result of complex interaction between various body systems and can be influenced by multiple factors, including lifestyle, diet, and genetics. Sad but true—there really is no miracle weight-loss diet where you can eat everything you want in unlimited quantities and have weight drop off. The bottom line is that you need to eat differently and convert your body to one that can burn fat for fuel rather than sugar. (You will learn more about becoming a fat burner, as opposed to a sugar burner, for your body's energy needs in Chapter 7.)

However, eating better doesn't necessarily mean eating less food. You can eat a LOT of the kinds of foods that boost your metabolism, make your body burn calories just to digest them, nurture your glands, tune up your endocrine system, and keep you full. So there is no need to be hungry all the time. You simply need to change the kinds of foods you eat, substituting healthier, "livelier" foods for "deadening," calorie-dense foods. What foods to eat are addressed in many other books about healthy eating, so I will not go into what specific foods to eat in this book. (However, you can read my book *The New Weight Loss Blueprint* to learn about fifteen superfoods I recommend as must-eats.)

CONFRONTING OLD EATING HABITS

When confronted with change, you have the opportunity to engage in a valuable practice to explore your inner workings—including your habits, emotions, physical self, and thoughts. For example, cutting down on sugar may expose various cravings and help you uncover how you might be "using" sweets to energize or soothe yourself without giving it much conscious thought. Use your yoga practice to become more sensitive to yourself and explore your innermost feelings and motives. You might discover why some part of you is resistant to change and, thus, why you're sabotaging your best efforts at weight loss. Once uncovered, you can go about healing it; awareness of the issue is the first step.

GETTING HEALTHY IS THE FIRST STEP TO WEIGHT LOSS

Weight loss is much easier when all your systems are working correctly, including your metabolic, pulmonary, muscular, and endocrine systems. That's why you need to aim for "healthy" before you can achieve "slim." Every system, gland, and organ has its own contribution to make it so your body can function optimally on the food you give it. When any of these systems are not functioning properly, the entire organism gets bogged down. You don't burn food properly for energy. The body produces hormones that cause you to store fat instead of burn it. Bones begin to lose strength because they are not challenged by stress from the muscles, and you end up in a downward spiral of decreasing health and vigor.

Because of the metabolic mechanics of weight loss, we want to have our digestive and endocrine systems functioning as efficiently as possible. If these systems are sluggish or not doing their job, the efficiency of processing food into energy for exercise (and for living) will be compromised and our ability to burn fat and turn calories into muscle will decrease.

So that's why it is so important that you understand the holistic nature of your own body/mind/spirit system. When you attempt to become as healthy as you can, you are not actually working against yourself to achieve your weight loss goals. Health should always come first, because one system impacts the functioning of the others. For example, if you eat the wrong foods and need to take acid-reducing medicine for heartburn, it's a sign that you're not digesting your food. If you're not digesting your food properly, you won't get all the nutrients your food has to offer. If you don't drink enough water and eat enough fiber, your intestines will be filled with impacted waste that hampers your absorption of nutrients. If you're not getting enough nutrients, you'll be hungry all the time. If you're hungry all the time, you're probably feeding yourself more to try to satisfy that hunger. The entire (dysfunctional) cycle goes on and on, and your body struggles to maintain the status quo and resists making the positive (outward) changes you so desire.

Every system affects another system in your body, and although each organ and gland has its own job to do, the important idea that I want to impart is that every part of you is interdependent on every other part. So breathing is not exclusive from stretching, or from digestion, or from strength, in creating an optimally functioning organism. All the systems must work together.

CHAPTER 5

How Yoga Affects the Glands and Organs

If you understand why overall health is important to weight loss, you'll have the motivation to work more effectively to not only normalize your weight, but also to extend your years of healthy and productive living.

The entire human body is made up of interdependent systems that exist in an extremely delicate balance. When the body needs to react to a certain situation, the system allows certain hormones to be released from those glands. Fortunately, even though we might abuse one of the systems, others will take over to some extent for a certain period of time. For example, if you're not getting the energy you need for your daily tasks from metabolizing the food you eat or assimilating the nutrients, the adrenals will be called on to produce more of the "fight or flight" hormone, adrenalin, to give an additional boost in energy. However, if the adrenals are called on too often to provide this extra energy, they will become exhausted. If you're not eating enough nutrient-rich foods you need for energy, again, the adrenals will have to work overtime.

THE CHANGES ARE MORE THAN COSMETIC

Anyone who has practiced yoga will understand how the asanas (postures) build strength, improve flexibility, increase mobility, and harmonize body and mind, relieving stress and aiding relaxation. However, the reasons behind our enhanced levels of health are less understood. Most of us feel better in general because our digestion improves, we are less prone to illness, we have more energy, and our bodies seem to function more efficiently. This is due to the effects that yoga has on our glands and internal organs. It's not just about what we can readily see, but what is going on inside us. Yoga is the only activity able to massage all the internal organs and glands of the body thoroughly and in a balanced way.

BREATHING

Pranayama (breathing) is the universal energy that sustains all life. When we inhale, every cell is supplied with energy, oxygen, and nutrients. When we exhale, waste and toxins are released. Establishing and maintaining yoga postures demands effective breathing. As we work into the postures, the lungs awaken and release their tension. Dormant lung tissue is reactivated, setting up more beneficial patterns of breathing deeply and fully. Many postures work specifically to open the chest and strengthen respiratory muscles. The heart and lungs are strengthened and able to perform their tasks more efficiently.

THE GLANDS' FUNCTION

The complex living functions of our body are controlled and monitored by a number of very important "ductless" glands. These are called endocrine glands. A person with a balanced endocrine system—which contains the pituitary gland, thyroid gland, adrenals, and sex glands—is generally happy, energetic, and strong. An unbalanced endocrine system results in depression, excess weight gain, sluggishness, and high levels of stress. The glands' main function is to generate and secrete hormones that help regulate your growth and metabolism, for reproductive purposes, and throughout pregnancy. Together, all act in close kinship with each other, as well as with our sympathetic nervous system. The brain controls many functions via the pituitary gland, the master gland of the body that regulates the secretion of hormones in all the other glands.

Different yoga postures work on different glands by increasing the blood supply to them; squeezing out the depleted, toxin-filled blood; and then allowing fresh blood to flood back in on release of the posture. The poses bring oxygen and nutrients, which are vital for healthy operation, to the glands. The glands of the immune system are also supported, enabling us to fight disease.

INTERNAL ORGANS

Other than those of the respiratory system mentioned above, the liver, kidneys, pancreas, brain, and reproductive organs are also massaged, stimulated, and toned, ridding them of toxins and improving their overall health and function. The pancreas, for instance, secretes insulin that helps regulate the levels of sugar in the blood. If it is dysfunctional, we may develop diabetes. Forward bends tone and stimulate the liver and kidneys. Adding a twist aids digestion as well as massages most of the other internal organs. Bridge pose can help stimulate the reproductive organs.

When the glands and internal organs function properly, then all the systems of the body work as they should. Everything in the body is connected to everything else, nothing exists without input from other systems, and everything has an effect on everything else. So with yoga, not only do the postures and lifestyle help make all the glands and organs healthy and more efficient, but you become more cognizant and sensitive to your body. You can be aware if something is not functioning properly and take action.

THE GLANDS AND ORGANS THAT YOGA AFFECTS

The glands and organs that yoga affects include:

Endocrine glands (the thyroid, adrenals, pineal, pituitary, pancreas, and hypothalamus)

Heart

Spleen

Stomach

Lungs

Liver/Gallbladder

Kidneys

Bladder

Large and Small Intestines

ENDOCRINE GLANDS AND THE HORMONES THEY PRODUCE

The endocrine glands secrete hormones that regulate various functions throughout the body. Endocrine glands release chemical messengers, or hormones, into the bloodstream to be transported to various organs and tissues. For instance, the pancreas secretes insulin, which allows the body to regulate levels of sugar in the blood. The thyroid gets instructions from the pituitary to secrete hormones that determine the pace of chemical activity in the body (the more hormone in the bloodstream, the faster the chemical activity; the less hormone, the slower the activity).

Hypothalamus

The hypothalamus is a small portion of the brain that is in very close proximity to the pituitary gland. It controls the pituitary hormones by releasing hormones that stimulate or inhibit their release. For example, the hypothalamus secretes gonadotropin-releasing hormone, which causes the production of gonado-tropins (follicle-stimulating hormone and luteinizing hormone) by the pituitary. It also produces corti-cotrophin-releasing hormone, thyrotropin-releasing hormone, and growth-hormone-releasing hormone.

The hypothalamus is responsible for sensing the amount of the hormone leptin in the bloodstream and instructing the body to burn sugar or fat for fuel. Leptin is a chemical messenger made in fat cells that speaks to the hypothalamus gland in the brain. When the hypothalamus becomes desensitized to leptin, it thereafter operates as if it "has no fat" in panic mode and continuously instructs the cells in one's body to burn sugar instead of fat for energy. In addition to the issue of weight gain that this causes, the constant burning of sugar for energy is unhealthy.

Pineal Gland

The pineal gland is a small gland located within the brain that secretes the hormone melatonin, which regulates the cycle of sleep and waking. In humans, as with all mammals, your biological clock resides in the suprachiasmatic nucleus of your brain (SCN), which is part of your hypothalamus. Based on signals of light and darkness, your SCN tells your pineal gland when it's time to secrete melatonin. It is exquisitely sensi-tive to cycles of light and darkness. Light comes in through your eyes and travels up your optic nerves to the rice-grain-sized SCN, which then interacts with many other regions of the brain. When you turn on a light at night, you immediately send your brain misinformation about the light-dark cycle. The only thing your brain interprets light to be is day. Believing daytime has arrived, your biological clock instructs your pineal gland to immediately cease its production of melatonin.[11]

Lack of sleep affects our ability to lose weight and has a lot to do with our nightly production of certain hormones. Here's how. The two hormones that are key in this process are ghrelin and leptin. Ghrelin is the "go" hormone that tells you when to eat, and when you are sleep-deprived, you have more ghrelin. Leptin is the hormone that tells you to stop eating, and when you are sleep deprived, you have less leptin. Thus, more ghrelin plus less leptin equals weight gain.[12]

Pituitary Gland

The pituitary is sometimes referred to as the "master gland" because it controls hormone functions such as temperature, thyroid activity, growth during childhood, urine production, testosterone production in males, and ovulation and estrogen production in females. In effect, the pituitary gland functions as our

---

11 Dr. Russel Reiter, *http://articles.mercola.com/sites/articles/ archive/2013/03/19/melatonin-benefits.aspx*

12 Michael Breus, PhD, *author of Beauty Sleep, Clinical Director, Arrow-head Health, Glendale, AZ, WebMD, 2012*

thermostat that controls all other glands responsible for hormone secretion. Your pituitary gland receives messages from another part of your brain, the hypothalamus, which has received messages from the environment or other areas of your body. For example, if one of your hormone levels gets too low, your hypothalamus will send a message via hormones to your pituitary gland. In response, your pituitary gland secretes hormones of its own and sends them through your bloodstream like little messengers. If all is going as it should, these hormones reach the gland that had not been producing enough of its own hormones. The hormones from your pituitary gland then stimulate new hormone production out of the misbehaving gland. If a gland is overproducing hormones, then your pituitary gland will send the message to lower hormone production.

Thyroid and Parathyroid Glands

The thyroid produces thyroxin and triiodothyronine, which are known to regulate metabolism. It also secretes calcitonin, which helps regulate calcium levels. Some of the other critical functions that the thyroid controls include body temperature, energy and fuel combustion, digestive enzymes, stomach acid production, fat and protein synthesis, metabolic rate, and synthesis and release of hormones that control bone and hair growth and skin rejuvenation.

Adrenal Glands

There are two adrenal glands, referred to as supra-renal glands, located on top of the kidneys. The adrenal glands are composed of two major components, the adrenal cortex and the adrenal medulla. The adrenal medulla secretes hormones, including both epinephrine and norepinephrine. The adrenal medulla increases available energy, heart rate, and metabolism. The hormones produced by the adrenal cortex are vital for life and include the glucocorticoids, mineralocorticoids, and some sex hormones like androgens and small amounts of estrogen.

Cortisol is also produced by your adrenal glands. This "stress hormone" helps regulate blood pressure and the immune system during a sudden crisis, whether a physical attack or an emotional setback. This helps you to tap into your energy reserves and increases your ability to fight off infection. Relentless stress can keep this survival mechanism churning in high gear, subverting the hormone's good intentions. Chronically high cortisol levels can cause sleep problems, a depressed immune response, blood sugar abnormalities, and abdominal weight gain.

Pancreas

Located between the stomach and the small intestine, the pancreas is both a gland and an organ, part of the digestive and endocrine system. As an endocrine gland, it produces several important hormones, including insulin, glucagon, and somatostatin. As an exocrine gland, it secretes pancreatic juice containing digestive enzymes that pass into the small intestine. These enzymes help in the breakdown of the carbohydrates, protein, and fat in the chyme, the pulpy acidic fluid consisting of gastric juices and partially digested food that passes from the stomach to the small intestine.

Here is an example of how the pancreas works in secreting hormones that control your blood sugar levels. Insulin and glucagon are hormones that work to regulate the level of sugar (glucose) in the body to keep it within a healthy range. The amount of glucose in your bloodstream and cells varies depending on what you've eaten, how much exercise your muscles are doing, and how active your body's cells are. These two hormones, insulin and glucagon, have the job of keeping tight control on the amount of glucose in your blood so that it doesn't rise or fall outside healthy limits. When someone has type 1 diabetes, they must give themselves insulin shots because their pancreas doesn't work and too much glucose in their blood causes "hyperglycemia."

If you eat a lot of sugar at any one time, your blood sugar goes way up and your body releases insulin to bring it down. To do this, insulin forces your body to store all that sugar in fat cells.

In the long term, a few things can happen. Your fat cells may begin to hold onto that energy a lot longer, making it even harder to lose weight and/or making it even easier for you to gain it. Those constant insulin spikes can cause something caused insulin resistance, which is basically the first step in type 2 (non-insulin-dependent) diabetes. Insulin resistance can be caused by medications, not taking enough insulin, diet choices, and illness. If left untreated, insulin resistance can cause an array of health complications, some of which can be fatal.

For these reasons, it is very important for your pancreas to continue secreting appropriate amounts of the substances (insulin and glucagon) to keep your body in balance.

Ovaries

Found only in women, these two small glands produce estrogen, progesterone, and inhibin. Estrogen and progesterone are the primary sex hormones responsible for many of the female secondary sex characteristics. Inhibin is a hormone that controls levels of follicle-stimulating hormone, which regulates egg development.

The ovaries are sensitive to the effects and changes of the endocrine, or hormonal, system. They respond to and produce their own hormones as needed by the body. In fact, the second major role of the ovary is to secrete the sex hormones (like estrogen and progesterone, which cause the typical female sex characteristics to develop and be maintained), and very small amounts of androgens. In addition, the ovaries also respond to FSH and LH, which are produced by the pituitary gland. FSH, or follicle-stimulating hormone, causes the estrogen level to rise and a group of egg follicles to grow each month. As one follicle becomes dominant and reaches maturity, the higher estrogen level will cause the LH (luteinizing hormone) to surge, triggering ovulation.

Testes

The testes, also known as testicles or male gonads, lie behind the penis in a pouch of skin called the scrotum. Found only in men, the testicles produce sperm and secrete testosterone, the primary hormone responsible for the male secondary sex characteristics. Testosterone decreases with age in men, and the loss of it can cause weight gain. Stress is another major factor that can affect testosterone production. By decreasing stress levels, you can decrease the hormone cortisol, which prevents the buildup of testosterone levels. Stress and cortisol buildup can be lowered by relaxation techniques (including pranayama breathing), yoga, or both.

THE TWO MAJOR PLAYERS IN THE WEIGHT LOSS GAME

Insulin plays an essential role in healthy body function, but an excess of it will make you fat. Too much insulin not only encourages your body to store unused glucose as fat, but also blocks the use of stored fat as an energy source. For these reasons, an abnormally high insulin level makes losing fat, especially around the abdomen, almost impossible.

Another hormone responsible for unwanted belly fat is cortisol. As mentioned above, cortisol is the hormone responsible for helping us deal with long-term stress, as compared to adrenalin (the "fight or flight" hormone), which is involved in the immediate response to stress. An elevated cortisol level destroys muscle fibers, suppresses immunity, affects memory and concentration, can weaken bone mineral density, and contributes to cancer. It can cause increased body fat, particularly around the abdomen, by adversely affecting blood sugar and insulin levels. High levels of cortisol are also very detrimental because they lead to other hormonal imbalances. Together, these two hormones (insulin and cortisol) will have you battling an insatiable appetite and craving carbs.

THE HORMONES YOGA STIMULATES TO HELP YOU LOSE WEIGHT

These hormones are all a part of our marvelous and complicated endocrine system, which controls weight, metabolism, sexual development, energy output, hair and bone growth, and other functions. They include:

Thyroid – (thyroxine and T3) Controls the rate at which muscle cells use energy.

Adrenaline – One of the functions of adrenaline is to break down fat stores and burn them. Some researchers believe that adrenaline can also decrease appetite.

Insulin and Glucagons – Fat-storing and fat-burning hormones that regulate the amount of blood sugar in your body at any one point.

Testosterone – Regulates fat production and builds lean muscle mass that assists in fat burning.

Human Growth Hormone (HGH) – Regulates how much fat instead of sugar gets burned for energy.

Insulin-like Growth Factor – A fat-burning hormone that gets stimulated by HGH and helps fuel your body between meals by releasing stored fat and sugar to create energy for functioning.

WHY HOW WELL YOU SLEEP IS IMPORTANT

Yoga is one of the best self-soothing techniques, such as meditation, relaxation, and exercise, to reduce stress and anxiety. By doing so, yoga decreases the output of hormones that the body naturally produces to combat stress by reducing the heart rate, lowering blood pressure, and easing respiration. Another interesting fact is that researchers have found significantly higher melatonin levels in experienced meditators in the period immediately following meditation. Melatonin is the "sleep" hormone, which, when the pineal gland is producing it in enough quantity, allows you to relax better.

Researchers have evaluated the effects of three months of Hatha Yoga practice and meditation on melatonin secretion. For three months, yoga group subjects practiced selected yoga postures for forty-five minutes and breathing exercises for fifteen minutes during the morning, and again for one hour in the evening daily. Results showed that yoga practice for only three months resulted in an improvement in cardiorespiratory performance and psychological profile. These observations suggest that yoga practices can be used to increase secretion of melatonin, which, in turn, is responsible for an improved sense of well-being. In other studies, it has been found that subjects trained in yoga can achieve a state of deep psycho-somatic relaxation associated with highly significant decrease in oxygen consumption within five minutes of practicing slow, rhythmic, and deep breathing, and corpse pose.[13]

The body uses sleep to repair itself, reset hormone levels, and prepare to function optimally the next day. Leptin levels rise all day and peak just before midnight, unless we eat late in the evening and/or don't get enough sleep, in which case leptin levels continue rising virtually all night. High leptin levels cause the hypothalamus to be unable to react to the leptin levels in the blood; the hypothalamus then acts as though leptin is low. We need to ensure that sufficient sleep occurs to bring leptin levels down to their daily lows before morning. If we don't do this, higher leptin levels in the morning will signal for our energy to be low and for fat to be stored, which is the opposite of what is desirable.[14]

---

13 *Pallav Sengupta, International Journal of Preventive Medicine, July 2012, http://www.ncbi.nlm.nih.gov/pmc/articles/PMC3415184/*
14 *Booklet: Becoming Leptin Sensitive, Editors, Healthy-Living.org*

CHAPTER 6

Introducing the Yoga Poses

With the hundreds of yoga poses that exist, how do you know which ones will be best for you? Here I'll not only introduce you to the poses that I think are most effective for weight loss, but I'll also explain why the poses will help you tune up your metabolic fat-burning system and thus help you lose weight faster. In addition, later on you'll see some sequences for yoga sessions that you can do at home.

These days, Hatha is most often used to describe the type of yoga that uses gentle, basic postures with rest between poses. A Hatha class will likely be a slow-paced stretch class with some simple breathing exercises and perhaps seated meditation. This is a good place to learn beginners' poses and relaxation techniques, and become comfortable with yoga. Many people try a Hatha class and love the relaxed feeling; others may decide that Hatha Yoga is too slow and meditative for them. If you fall in the latter category, you will want to try Vinyasa or Power Yoga for a different and more active, intense experience.

Vinyasa Yoga, in which movement is synchronized to the breath, is a term that covers a broad range of yoga classes. This style is sometimes also called "flow yoga" because of the smooth way that the poses run together and become like a dance. The breath becomes an important component because often the teacher will instruct you to move from one pose to the next on an inhale or an exhale. Vinyasa is literally translated from Sanskrit as meaning "connection." In terms of yoga asana, we can interpret this not only as a connection of all the poses because of the way one pose flows into the next, but also between movement and breath.

Whether you choose to string the poses together in a "vinyasa," or simply do each pose sequentially as part of a series, is up to you, based on your energy level and experience.

You should spend at least one minute doing each pose. Take a look at the picture before you start and try to emulate the way it looks using a mirror.

If you are just starting out with yoga, do each of the poses one time per session, which will be about twenty minutes, and complete about six sessions of the beginner poses before you start to attempt the yoga sequences. The only exception to this is the Relaxation Sequence, which can be done by anyone, anytime. The average amount of time that should be spent in any one pose is five deep inhalations and exhalations. If you feel like it would be beneficial to spend more time in a flexibility pose, for example, you can do so, but make sure your treat both sides of your body equally. If you have difficulty holding a more challenging pose for that long, definitely come out of it earlier. Perhaps a good slogan to remember would be, "Practice to practice another day." In other words, be gentle, somewhat cautious, and allow yourself to be guided by how it feels. Only you can determine the pace of your practice. Many times I have overdone my yoga practice in a too-advanced class, allowing my ego to get carried away and dictate my degree of performance, and have ended up suffering the next day because I pushed too hard.

You can break up your yoga practice into different segments if you like; for example, practicing the more energizing Stamina Sequence in the morning and the Relaxation Sequence at night before bed. You can string two sequences together or mix up the poses in one session.

YOGA POSES FOR RELAXATION

STANDING FORWARD BENDS (UTTANASANA)

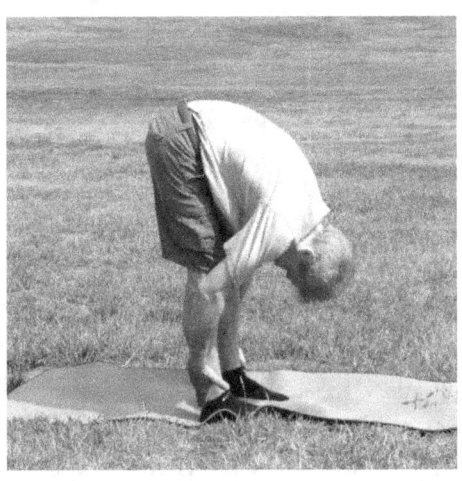

Often used as a transition between poses, this pose has many benefits when practiced by itself. The posture stretches the hamstrings, thighs, and hips, and is thought to relieve stress, fatigue, and mild depression.

As when you start any pose, be mindful of your body's limitations and be gentle and compassionate with yourself, even if you feel you should be able to go further. Listen to your body, breathe, and ease into the stretch.

Forward bending stretches out the back side of the body completely, from the Achilles tendons to the top of the neck. This stretch creates spinal decompression using gravity alone, and it is a very gentle and safe way to add more space to the intervertebral discs. This is important because as you age the weight of the body tends to make the discs bulge slightly, and if they bulge enough to impinge on any of the spinal nerves, the result is often very painful. Any kind of natural spinal decompression is valuable, but it must be done gently to avoid any damage to ligaments and muscles. If your goal is to de-stress in the pose, it's best done with the knees slightly bent.

An important thing to remember with forward bending is to attempt to keep the spine relatively flat and bend from the hips rather than from the waist. The goal is to stretch the hamstring muscles and not strain the muscles in the lower back. When starting out, you may be so tight that you will feel any attempt at a forward bend all the way from the back of your knees to your neck. As you get a little more flexible, you'll be able to tell which muscles are getting the greatest stretch and you'll be able to adjust the pose accordingly.

Forward bends can be done standing or sitting, with straight legs or slightly bent legs, narrow stance or hip-width or wider. With the wide-leg forward bend, you may also want to try adding a small spinal twist by stretching the right hand over to the left foot and vice versa. This twist stimulates the adrenals, stretches the intercostal muscles (which makes deep breathing easier), and compresses and stretches different parts of the colon and small intestines. Forward bending even helps in digestion by gently compressing and massaging the abdomen. Standing forward bends also help digestion by relieving some of gravity's weight on the intestines.

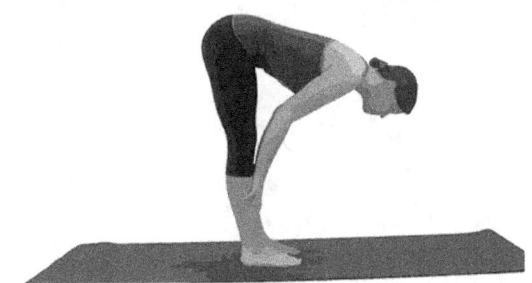

Variation 1 – Hands on shins. For complete beginners, even this might be too intense, so a modified version is to put your hands on the seat of a chair to support the weight of your upper body and just hang out there for a minute or two. As always, don't forget to relax the back of the neck and breathe.

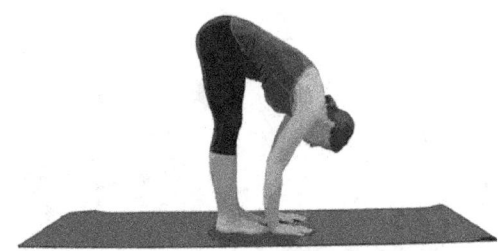

Variation 2 – Hands on floor. As your hamstrings get a little more flexible, you will be able to drop down further. Remember to point the top of your head toward the floor, relaxing the back of your neck, and hinge from the hips rather than the waist.

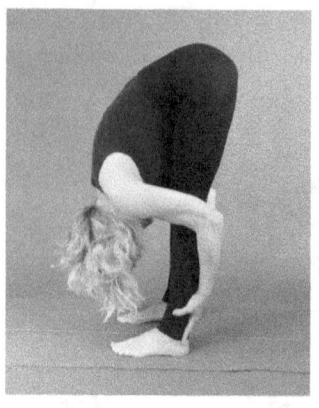

Variation 3 – Forearms tucked behind calves. Try to flatten your torso along your thighs, even if you have to bend your knees slightly to get your forearms tucked around the back of your calves. Then, using your arm strength to hold your torso on your thighs, begin to straighten your legs by pushing your knees back, but do not lock your knees out. Be sure you are pointing the top of your head toward the floor, so you don't tighten and crunch the back of the neck. Breathe!

SEATED FORWARD BEND (PASCHIMOTTANASANA)

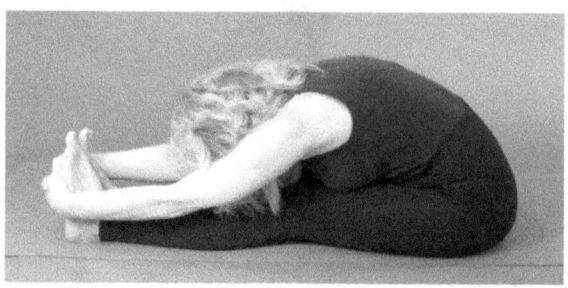

Variation 4 – Boost circulation with this calming forward bend that helps a distracted mind unwind. The pose is performed by sitting on the floor with the legs straight in front of you and feet flexed. Bend

forward at the waist and reach the arms straight ahead, relaxing into the pose while keeping the knees straight. If forward bending gets easy for you, flex your feet and wrap your hands around your soles.

SIDE BENDS

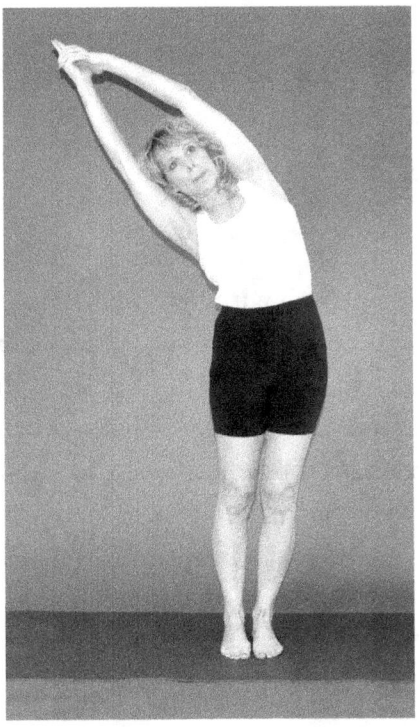

Side bends are great for waking up the entire torso and trimming excess fat from around the waist and the hip area, because side bends work one side of the body while stretching the other. Side bending makes deep breathing easier while in the pose and thereby makes your everyday breathing more efficient. The pose expands your breathing capacity by stretching the intercostal muscles between the ribs and helps increase lymph flow to eliminate toxins by stimulating the areas with the most lymph glands, including the armpit and groin areas.

How to do it:

Stretch both arms over the head, clasping the hands together and extending the index fingers out. Keep the elbows drawn in to the side of the head and keep your arms as straight as possible. Use your back muscles to move your upper arms farther back behind the ears if you can.

After you reach up with both arms, pull your shoulders down and away from your ears so your shoulders are not hunched up around your ears. Inhale, then slowly on an exhale, start dropping your upper body to the side. Keep your chest open to the front of the room, as if you were being held between two giant sheets of glass, so your body stays on one plane. It's okay if you cannot go over very far to the side; just a few inches will do for a start. If you feel comfortable there, you can always go a little farther.

Keep your face either looking straight ahead or look up slightly toward the ceiling if your neck remains comfortable. Keep breathing here for thirty seconds, then come back to upright and side bend on the other side. It will feel so good that you'll probably want to do it again on each side!

PLOW POSE (HALASANA)

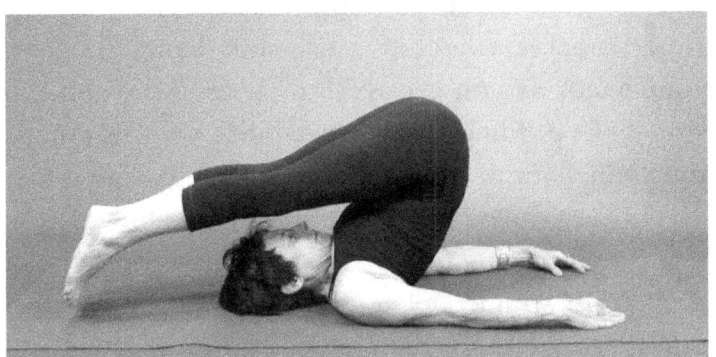

The plow pose is essentially an inverted forward bend. All inverted poses are beneficial for sending more blood to the brain and giving your circulatory system a rest by reversing the force that your heart must struggle against much of the time (gravity). The plow pose is an especially important inversion because it increases circulation to and stimulates the thyroid, adrenal, and pituitary glands.

How to do it:

Lying on your back, place your hands palms down on the floor with your thumbs just under your hips. Bring both legs up toward the ceiling (one at a time or together), and using your abdominal muscles, attempt to bring your feet up to your forehead while still keeping your hips on the floor.

If you can do this without difficulty, simply swing your legs over your head again with a little more controlled force to elevate your hips and bring your feet toward the floor beyond your head. You can either support your hips with your hands or grasp your hands as you gently allow your entire spine to stretch. Depending on your flexibility, your feet might touch the floor or not, and it's completely okay if they don't. Keep your chin tucked into the hollow of your throat to stimulate the thyroid gland and protect your neck from strain. Do not turn your head to either side unless you're very sure you can do that without injuring yourself.

Some yogis like to fold a thick blanket to about two inches high and place it under the shoulders so your head and neck are lower than your shoulders, allowing the neck to be in a more relaxed, less extreme position. Try it to see if it works better for you.

BACKWARD BENDS

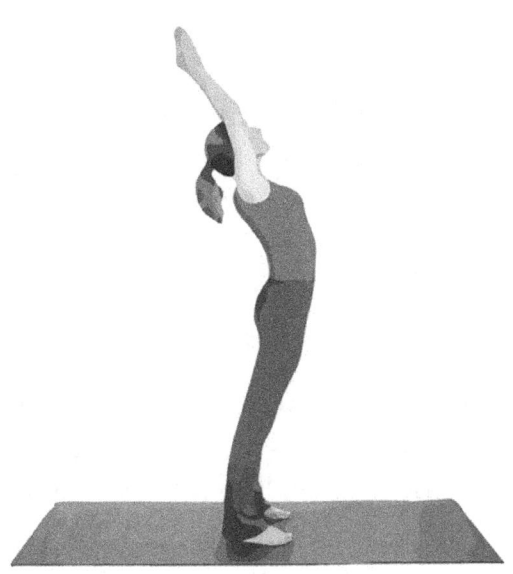

Backward bends include standing back bending, Cobra, and Bow poses. The benefits of back bending poses include stretching out the front of the abdomen and waking up the deep postural muscles that make up our core, while strengthening the back muscles that allow us to remain upright. Keeping these muscles strong will protect the back against strain from lifting, because we will be "practicing" using the muscles in a controlled way. Back bending opens up the hip flexor muscles as well (the tight muscles in the front of the body where the legs meet the torso), which tend to chronically shorten from sitting at your desk, in the car, and watching TV. Most people have very weak hamstring (back of the thigh), gluteus (buttocks), and lower back muscles, and overly strong quadriceps muscles in the front of the leg, which creates imbalances that lead to injury.

Poses that involve backward stretching create circulation to the groin area and stimulate lymphatic drainage, allowing you to eliminate toxins that contribute to cellulite and the puckered skin look, which are really just deposits of fat and toxins.

How to do it:

When practicing this posture, squeeze the gluteus muscles in the buttocks, stretch up through the chest, drop your shoulders, and keep lifting the heart area. Think of this as more of a "chest lift" than a "back bend," then drop your arms back as far as you can behind your ears and look up. Pull in your stomach muscles and keep your hips engaged, hugging the muscles into the bones. And breathe.

COBRA POSE (BHUJANGASANA)

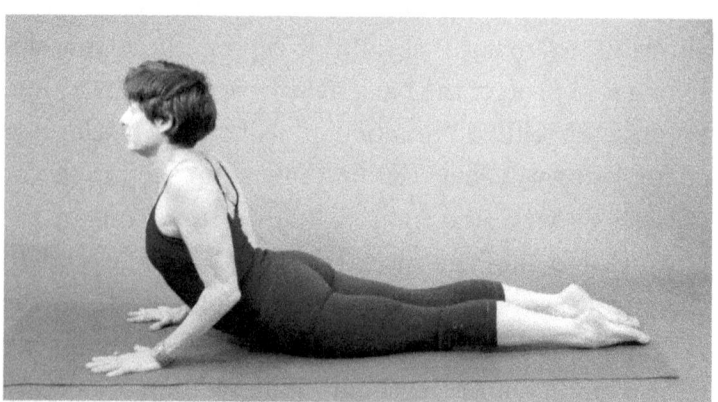

Cobra Pose resembles a cobra that is ready to strike. It stimulates the kidneys and adrenals and strengthens the organs of the digestive system. Besides facilitating weight loss, it makes the spine more flexible and opens up the chest for better breathing. Cobra counteracts the tendency that some people have for rounded shoulders and sunken chests, and it improves posture significantly. Some yoga teachers say that the Cobra Pose helps you to overcome fear, expand your heart, and experience more love in your life. Cobra will definitely help you develop more confidence and self-esteem.

How to do it:

1. Lying prone with the tops of the feet on the floor, place your hands flat on the floor beside your chest. Hug your elbows into your sides, using your arm and back muscles, and arch up as far as you comfortably can. It is not important that you straighten your elbows. Keep your hipbones on the floor and keep pressing your shoulders down and away from your ears. You can look upward or straight ahead if looking up causes any neck discomfort. Take three to five deep inhales and exhales here, then release and lower.

1. If this creates any tightness in the lower back, do the counter-stretch called Child's Pose. Push your body back and sit your buttocks on your heels with your knees slightly open so your body can nestle in between your thighs, and with your arms

by your side, rest your head on the floor.

CHILD'S POSE (BALASANA)

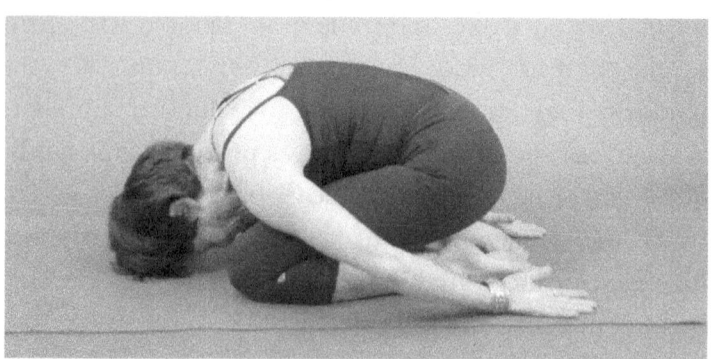

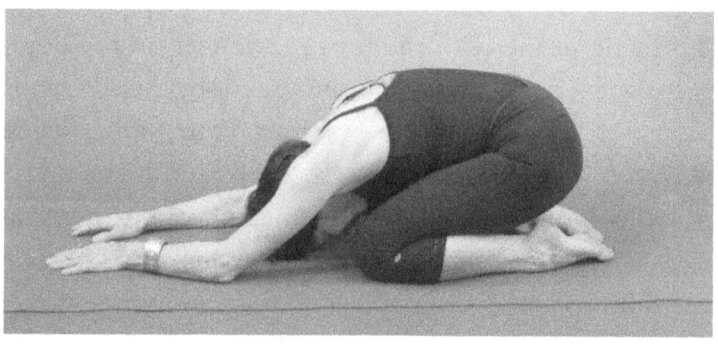

SEATED SPINAL TWIST (ARDHA MATSYENDRASANA)

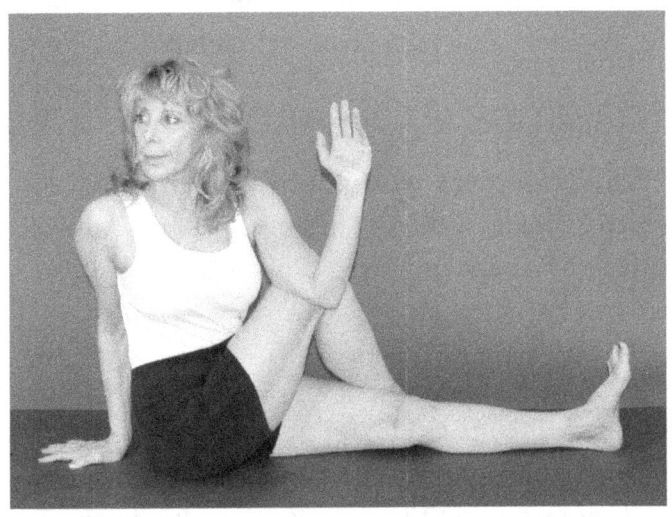

Spinal twists are dynamic poses that awaken the torso, stimulating the digestive system and energizing the spine. There are so many wonderful benefits to twisting and wringing your spine to give it length and suppleness. Not only do spinal twists give articulation to every vertebra, but they also keep the discs in between the vertebrae spongy and lubricated. Since there are so many nerves running up and down the spine, spinal twists both energize and sooth the nervous system and trigger deep relaxation, especially when coupled with deep breathing. Spinal twists also tone the muscles in your abdominal region and stimulate your entire digestive system. By stretching the complete length of the spine, including your neck, you address the area where you might hold a lot of stress.

(If you don't already know it, stress plays a big part in your metabolic balance; it inhibits the ability of the immune system to protect the body, slows wound healing, adds fat to your torso and belly area, and may even diminish muscle strength.)

There are a variety of ways to do spinal twists, which include sitting, standing, and lying down. I'll include a variety and you can choose which one(s) you like best.

How to do it:

1. Sit with your left leg stretched out in front of you, with the right leg bent at the knee and the right foot resting on the outside of the left knee.

2. Place your right hand behind the base of your spine, and lifting the left arm up and over the bent right knee, use your left elbow to push against the outside of the right knee to facilitate the twisting pose.

3. Inhale as you lift the crown of your head up toward the ceiling, and exhale as you twist to the right, sending your gaze behind you.

4. Use your straight right arm to support the spine.

5. Inhaling, stretch up. Exhaling, twist. Do this three more times. If you want to loosen up your neck a little bit as you are twisting, lift your face toward the ceiling and then drop your chin down to your shoulder. Repeat, then release and switch sides. Keep breathing.

SEATED SPINAL TWIST VARIATION

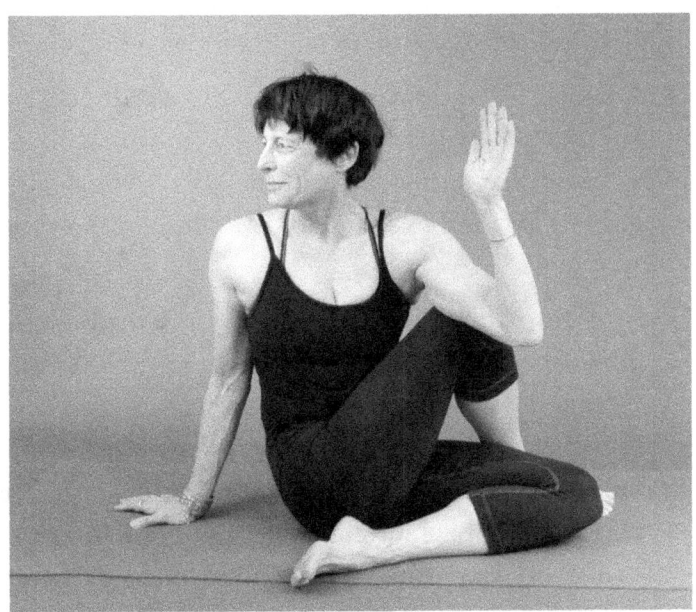

How to do it:

1. Sit with your feet on the floor and knees bent. Place your left foot under your right leg to the outside of your right hip. Put the outside of the left leg on the floor. Step the right foot over the left leg onto the floor outside your left hip.

2. Exhale and twist toward the right. Put the right hand against the floor behind your right buttock and set your left upper arm on the outside of your right thigh near the knee.

3. Press the right foot into the floor and lengthen the front torso. Sit tall, lean the upper torso back slightly, and continue to lengthen the spine.

4. You can turn your head in one of two directions: continue the twist of the torso by turning it to the right, or counter the twist of the torso by turning it left and looking over the left shoulder at the right foot.

5. With every inhalation, lift a little more through the upper chest, pushing the fingers against the floor to help. Twist a little more with every exhalation. Be sure to distribute the twist evenly throughout the entire length of the spine; don't concentrate it in the lower back. Remain in the pose for three to five breaths, then release with an exhalation, return to the starting position, and repeat to the left for the same length of time.

BOUND ANGLE POSE (BADDHA KONASANA)

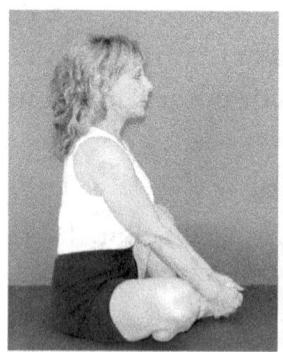 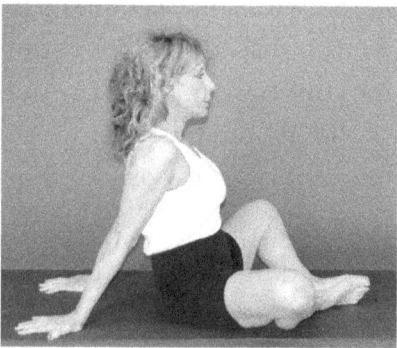

Bound Angle Pose is a powerful hip opener that lets you practice letting go in an area that is chronically tight for almost everyone, in an easy relaxed posture with your feet together in front of you and your knees bent out to the sides. By allowing the earth to support you in this pose, you can relax completely and let gravity do the work.

How to do it:

1. Start seated with your legs straight out in front of you. Exhale deeply and bend your knees while you move your heels toward your sit bones. Continue your exhale as you place the soles of your feet together and drop your knees toward the mat as far as they drop naturally, which might not be very far if you are extremely tight in your inner thighs and groin.

2. Inhale and lengthen your spine toward the ceiling as you grasp each hand around each corresponding ankle, pulling your heels as close to your pelvis as possible. Exhale deeply as you ensure your pelvis is in a neutral position, neither jutting forward nor rolled back.

3. Inhale deeply as you slide your shoulder blades down your back and lengthen the front of your torso to open the chest. Exhale deeply.

4. Hold the pose for up to three minutes, concentrating on maintaining symmetry in your body

positioning and your breath, with the depth of the inhales matching the depth of the exhales. Note which side of your body seems to be tighter or looser.

5. Release the pose on an exhale, moving your knees away from the floor and straightening your legs into your original seated position.

Note: If your inner thighs are so tight that you curl up like a shrimp when you open your knees, modify the pose by placing your hands behind your hips and sitting up as straight as possible. Find a position that you can hold for a few minutes and simply breathe, allow your knees to drop down, and open up your groin. Hello, inner thighs!

RECLINING BOUND ANGLE POSE
(SUPTA BADDHA KONASANA)

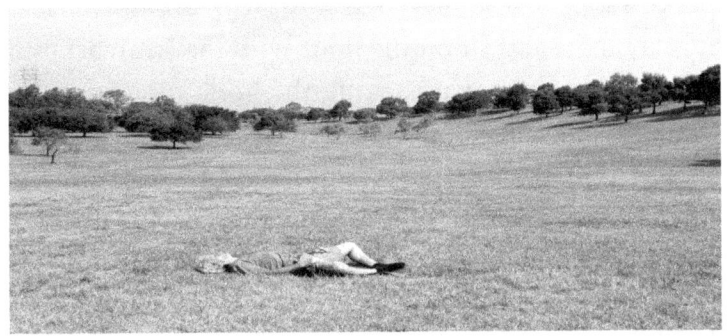

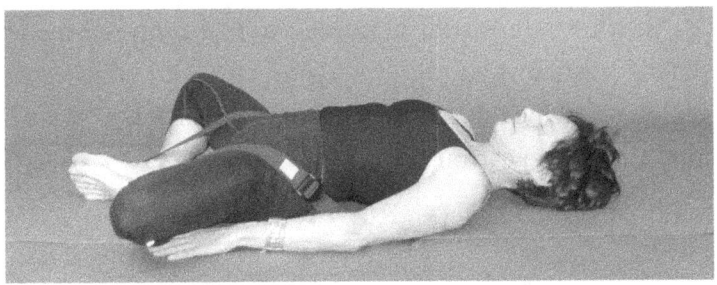

Another Bound Angle modification is to keep the soles of your feet together and your knees open to the sides, then lie down on your back. While most males have no issue sitting with their knees open, lying down in this position can be quite different. Just breathe and let your groin muscles relax and allow the adductor muscles in your inner, upper thigh to lengthen.

Another great way to do this pose is with a yoga strap around the waist, (thus the "bound" name) and looped around the feet so that they don't slide away from the body while you are reclining, since your arms are not long enough to hold your feet in. To do this, make a loop with your yoga strap with about two feet of play in it, and sit on the floor with the strap around the back of your waist. Bring the heels to your groin while sitting and loop the strap over the top of both feet so that the loop goes around your feet (over the ankles) and around your waist. Tighten the strap as far as you can comfortably tighten it, so that it keeps your feet close to your body without your having to hold them, then slowly lie down onto your back.

Another supported variation is to lie on a bolster placed vertically along your spine and put pillows or blocks under each of the knees to contain the stretch and allow relaxation with the knees open.

HAPPY BABY POSE (ANANDA BALASANA)

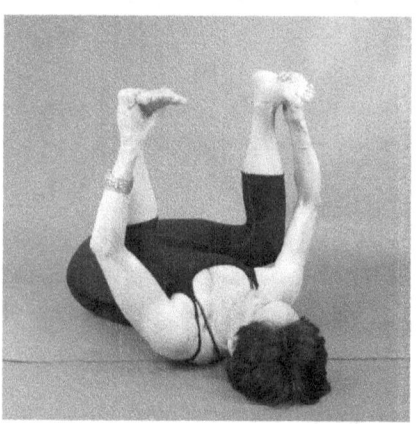

This is an easy-to-do hip opener pose, and it results in a very relaxing yet thorough stretch for the lower back. Bring your knees into your chest, opening your knees wide so that they point toward your armpits, grab the outside of your soles with your hands, and lift the bottom of your feet toward the ceiling. Try to flatten your tailbone back onto the floor, lengthening the spine, so you don't curl up like a shrimp while doing this pose.

LEGS UP THE WALL POSE (VIPARITA KARANI)

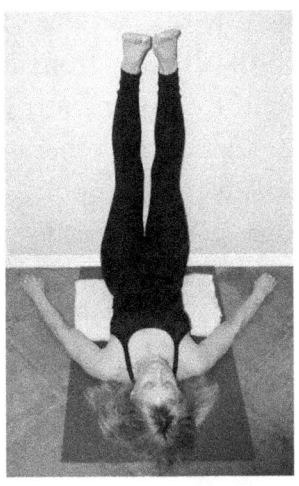

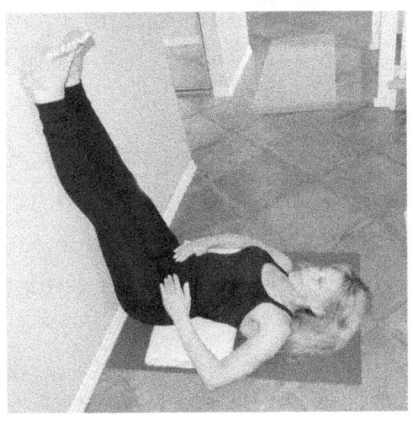

This pose is a powerhouse in disguise—a restorative pose that gently but effectively helps to bring more blood to the heart and brain while assisting lymph flow. The pose is almost magic in its ability to relax you. For support you'll need one or two thickly folded blankets or a firm round bolster.

How to do it:

1. Start by sitting with your side to the wall, about six inches away, with your knees bent. Lie on your side with your head away from and your sit bones facing the wall. Roll over onto your back, lifting one bent leg and then the other up the wall. If you are using a blanket as support, you can lift your hips with your feet against the wall and slide the blanket under your hips, experimenting a little with the placement so that the front of your abdomen faces squarely up toward the ceiling, rather than causing your abdomen to collapse and elongating the lower back.

2. After adjusting the support under your hips with your legs bent and your feet against the wall, straighten out your legs.

3. If you're stiff, the support can be lower and farther from the wall, making less of an acute angle; if you're more flexible, use a higher support that is closer to the wall. Your distance from the wall also depends on your height—if you're shorter, move closer to the wall; if taller, move farther from the

wall. Experiment with the position of your support until you find the placement that works for you, as you need to be able to relax. Your sit bones don't need to be right against the wall; they should drop down into the space between the support and the wall. The front of your torso should gently arch from the pubis to the top of the shoulders. If the front of your torso seems flat, then you've probably slipped back a bit and off your support. Bend your knees, press your feet into the wall, lift your pelvis off the support a few inches, and tuck the support a little higher up under your pelvis, then lower your pelvis onto the support again.

4. Lengthen your neck by releasing the base of your skull away from your shoulders (you can use your hands to do this) and soften your throat. Slide your shoulder blades away from the spine and release your hands and arms out to your sides, palms up.

5. Relax your feet and legs, with just enough tension to hold them vertically in place. Release your belly and soften your heart area.

6. Stay here anywhere from five to fifteen minutes. To come out of the pose, bend your knees and push your feet against the wall to lift your pelvis off the support. Then slide the support away, lower your pelvis to the floor, and turn onto your side. Stay on your side for a few breaths, then come up to sitting. (See photo next page.)

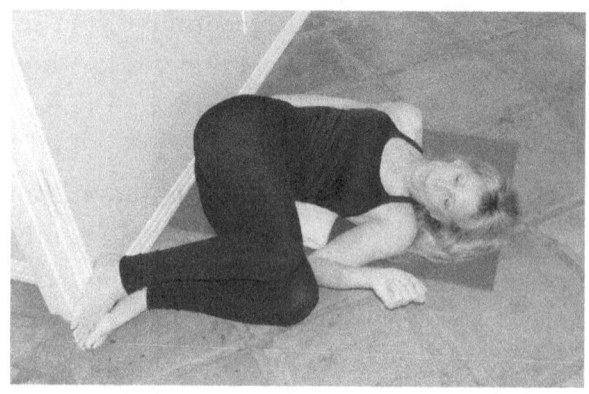

EXTENDED PUPPY POSE (UTTANA SHISHOSANA)

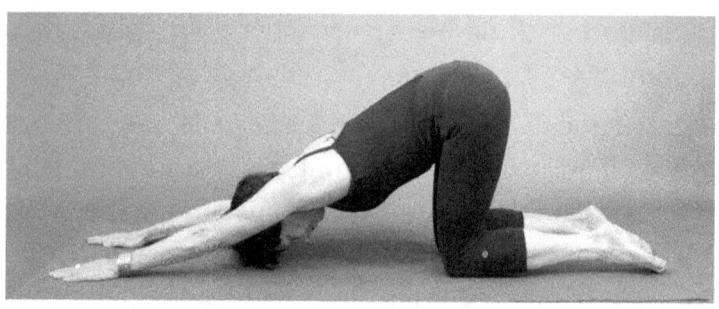

A variation of child's pose with a refreshing and heart-opening effect, this mild inversion pose can help to counter our tendency to curl forward or slouch the shoulders.

How to do it:

1. From Downward Facing Dog, drop your knees onto the mat, placing the tops of the feet on the mat. Keep the arms extended out in front of you, palms down. Walk your hands forward a few inches. Take a breath.

2. As you exhale, push your buttocks back toward your heels a few inches and drop your chest down toward the floor. It probably will not touch the floor, and that's fine.

3. Drop your forehead to the floor and let your neck relax. Keep a slight curve in your lower back. To feel a nice long stretch in your spine, press the hands down and stretch through the arms while pulling your hips back toward your heels. If your body tends to pull your arms back and lessen the stretch, creep your fingers forward a few inches and feel the armpits and latissimus muscles open up.

4. Breathe into your back, feeling the spine lengthen in both directions. Hold for thirty seconds to a minute, then release your buttocks down onto your heels and rest in Child's Pose for a minute, then repeat.

THREAD THE NEEDLE POSE

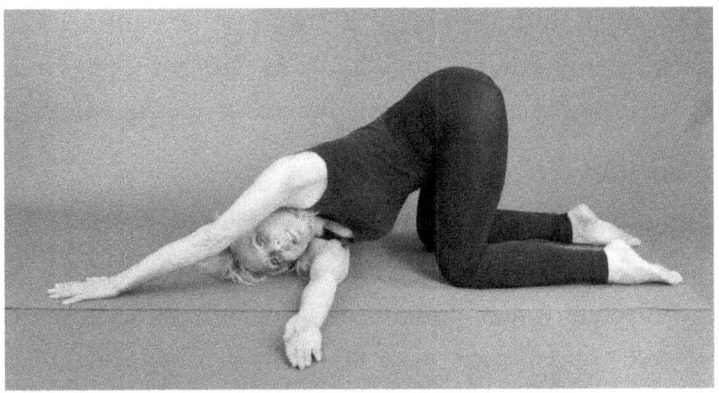

Thread the Needle Pose is a shoulder-releasing yoga posture that is suitable for most students, including beginners. This pose provides a lot of relief if you have stiffness and pain in your back, shoulders, or neck. Thread the Needle offers a number of variations to suit your level of flexibility.

This posture, while a bit complicated to get into, will give you a great stretch through the back and shoulders. It releases the tension that is commonly held in the upper back and between the shoulder blades. It also requires a gentle twisting motion that can help stretch and loosen the muscles in the lower back. If you are dealing with chronic shoulder or back pain, this posture can help gently loosen the muscles and relieve tension, but be cautious since the opportunity to overstretch is present.

Caution: Avoid practicing this pose if you have a recent or chronic injury to your knees, shoulders, or neck. Those with back injuries or degenerative disk disease should approach this pose with caution and should only attempt to practice it under the guidance of an experienced and knowledgeable instructor.

How to do it:

1. Begin on your hands and knees. Place your wrists directly under your shoulders and your knees directly under your hips. Point your fingertips to the top of your mat. Place your shins and knees

hip-width apart. Center your head in a neutral position and soften your gaze downward.

2. On an exhalation, slide your right arm underneath your left arm with your palm facing up. Let your right shoulder come all the way down to the mat. Rest your right ear and cheek on the mat, then gaze toward your left.

3. Keep your left elbow lifting and your hips raised. Do not press your weight onto your head; instead, adjust your position so most of the weight is on the side of your upper arm and shoulder.

4. Let your upper back broaden. Soften and relax your lower back. Breathe deeply and allow the tension in your shoulders, arms, and neck to drain away.

5. Hold for up to one minute. To release, press through your left hand and gently slide your right hand out. Return to Table Pose. Then repeat the pose on the opposite side for the same length of time.

Since Thread the Needle is a calming position, it's important to make whatever modifications you need to feel comfortable, safe, and supported in the pose. To lighten or deepen the intensity of the pose, try these simple changes:

If the pose hurts your kneecaps, fold your mat under your knees.

For a deeper shoulder stretch, come into the full pose. Then, bring the arm that is out in front supporting you (the arm that is not doing the "threading"), behind your body and rest the back of that hand on your lower back. Your lower arm should remain on the floor with your palm facing up.

PIGEON POSE

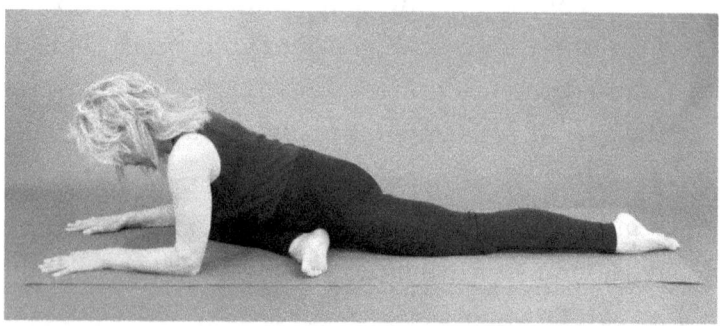

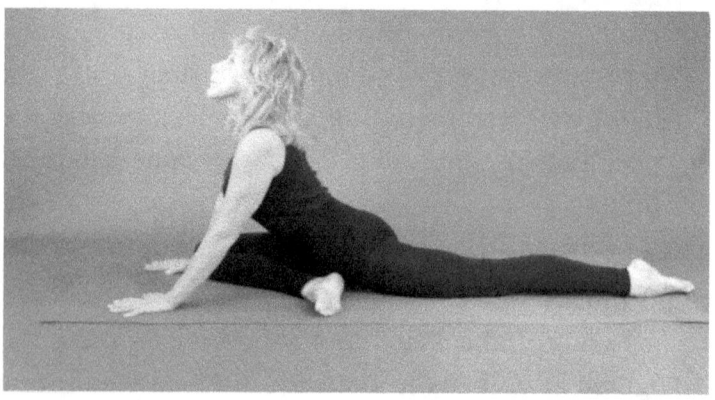

This pose is a massively effective hip opener that releases tension from an area where most of us are very tight but few of us ever want to go through the discomfort that it takes to release that tension. If you can ease into this pose and stay here for a few minutes, breathing deeply and letting go, you can integrate a lot of emotional negativity, because a lot of emotions seem to get stored in the hip and buttock area. Be very gentle and compassionate with yourself in this pose, as it is well worth the effort involved.

How to do it:

1. From Downward Facing Dog, step your right foot forward and over to your left hand, with the side of the foot below the wrist and the sole facing to the left.

2. Sit down onto your right hip, extending the left leg straight back behind you with the top of the knee pointing down into the floor and the top of the left sole on the floor.

3. Lower your torso onto the right thigh, with your knee either in the middle of your chest or pointing toward your right shoulder. Be sure you are sitting on your hip and not on top of your right leg, as this can be hard on your knee.

4. Rest here, either on your elbows with the palms down, breathing deeply and relaxing, or lower your entire body down on top of the thigh and rest with your head on the floor.

5. Arms can be brought back by the sides of the body to relax the shoulders or extended out in front of the body.

CAT TO COW POSE (MARJARYASANA)

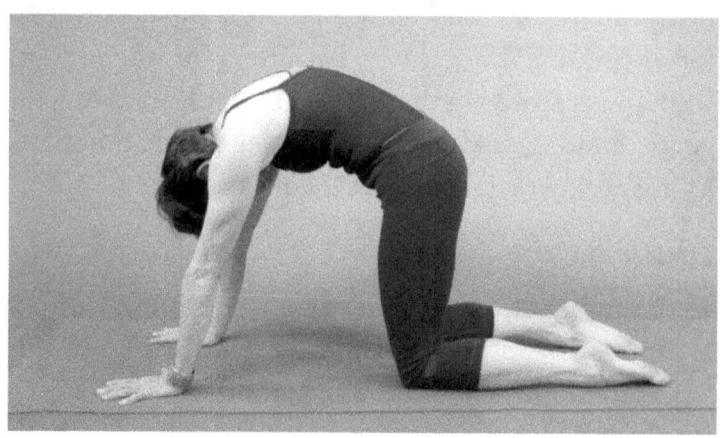

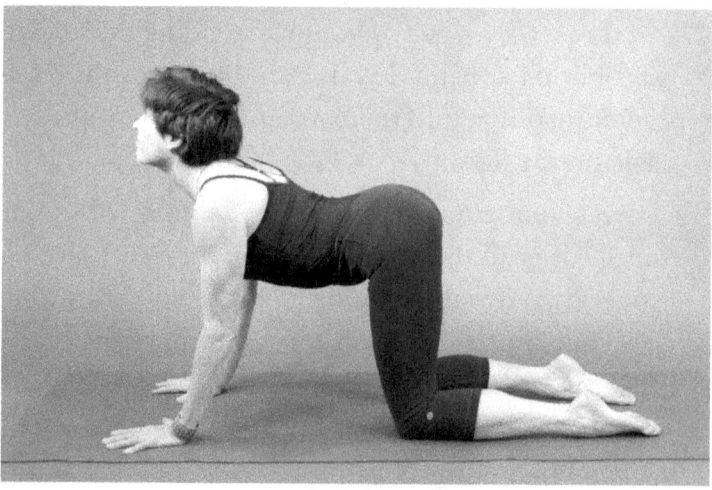

A wonderful way to start off any yoga practice is with Cat to Cow Pose. Often abbreviated as Cat-Cow, the combination of these two poses helps warm up your spine and relieves back and neck tension after a long day. It's a wonderful addition to your home practice or a perfect way to loosen up before a studio class.

How to do it:

1. Begin with your hands and knees on the floor. Make sure your knees are under your hips and your wrists are under your shoulders. Begin in a neutral spine position with your back flat and your abs engaged. Take a big, deep inhale.

2. On the exhale, round your spine up toward the ceiling and imagine you're pulling your belly button up toward your spine, really engaging your abs. Tuck your chin toward your chest and release your neck. This is your cat-like shape.

3. On your inhale, un-arch your back, let your belly relax, and go loose. Lift your head and tailbone up towards the sky—without putting any unnecessary pressure on your neck. This is the Cow portion of the pose.

4. Continue flowing back and forth, arching then flattening, from Cat Pose to Cow Pose, and connect your breath to each movement—inhale for Cow Pose and exhale on Cat Pose as you contract your stomach muscles.

5. Repeat for about ten rounds, or until your spine is warmed up.

SEATED HEAD TO KNEE POSE (JANUSIRSASANA)

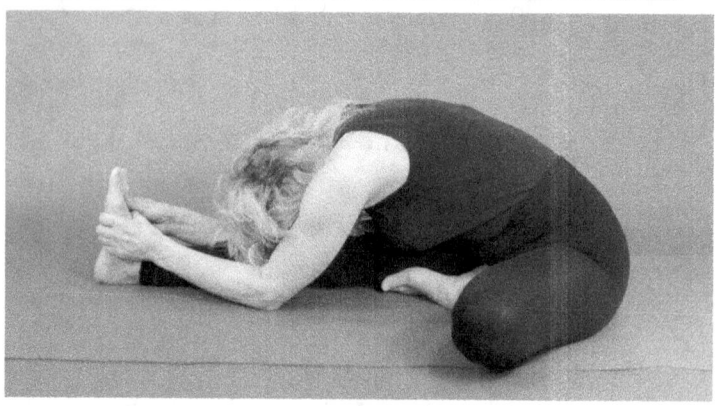

Relaxing, and allowing a deeper stretch than Seated Forward Bend, Seated Head to Knee Pose is a forward bend variation that can help boost blood flow and release tension.

How to do it:

1. Sitting on the floor with both legs in front of you, bend the left leg at a ninety-degree angle while you keep the right leg extended, placing the sole of the left foot touching the inner thigh of the extended right leg.

2. Stretch up, lifting the arms, and, hinging at the hip rather than the waist, bend over the extended leg and reach for your foot. Hold for sixty seconds, breathing deeply, and then repeat with the left leg extended. (Use a towel looped over the foot if you cannot reach it).

3. For a greater stretch in the rib and waist area, take the opposite hand to the outside of the extended leg. Remember to keep bending from the hip, flattening out your body along your thigh as you get more flexible, and reaching out with the crown of your head, face down toward your leg, so as not to scrunch up your neck.

CORPSE POSE (SAVASANA)

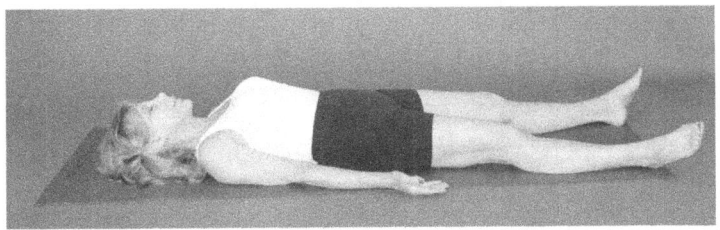

Most yoga practices end with several minutes spent in this pose, and it can easily be the most calming part of the whole session. The pose puts the body totally at ease by emphasizing complete relaxation. Corpse Pose triggers the body's "relaxation response," a state of deep rest that slows the breathing and lowers the blood pressure while quieting the nervous system. It is the ideal way to finish your practice because, in this relaxed yoga pose, you simply lie back and practice letting go. (Hint: It can be harder than it seems, because a corpse doesn't think about its "to-do" list, what's for dinner, or how it might have missed something on the latest P&L report.)

This pose is done at the end of the yoga session to allow the body to rest completely and regenerate, reaping the benefits from all the stretching, breathing, strengthening, and balancing that preceded it. You should always try to finish your yoga session with the Corpse Pose, even if you only have time for a few minutes of it.

How to do it:

1. Start seated on the mat with your legs bent and feet flat on the floor. Inhale deeply and then exhale, leaning back onto your forearms and slightly lifting your pelvis off the mat. Place the sacrum flat on the mat by tucking the tailbone toward the foot of the mat. Deeply inhale and slowly extend one leg, then the other, as you soften the groin and turn the feet slightly outward. Exhale deeply as you soften your lower back and feel your body sink gently onto the mat.

2. Inhaling, use your hands to lift the base of your skull away from your neck as you soften the muscles in the back of the neck. Exhale deeply as you broaden the base of your skull and wiggle your body around a bit to ensure that it feels symmetrical on the mat.

3. Deeply inhale and reach both arms toward the ceiling as you rock your body slightly side to side to broaden your back against the mat. Deeply

exhale and release your arms to the mat, turning the thumbs slightly outward and resting the backs of the hands on the mat.

4. Deeply inhale and then exhale while you concentrate on softening your tongue, your facial muscles, your scalp, and the skin on your forehead. Close your eyes and let them sink back into your skull; allow your brain to settle and do the same.

5. For the first minute or so, focus on your breathing. Breathe deeply and slowly, being mindful of each inhalation and exhalation. Deeply inhale, then completely relax and let the exhale flow out. Extend your exhalations by a second or two, making them longer than your inhalations. Pause slightly after each deep exhalation, languishing in this moment of stillness and quiet. Inhale deeply and breathe with your whole body, feeling the breath move the belly, and slightly rock the hips, shoulders, and spine. Feel the breath filter through every muscle and organ in your body, calming and soothing every cell. Exhale deeply, once again feeling it in every cell.

6. Now just begin to let go. Do not focus on the breath; allow it to become soft and natural, and simply observe where it goes. Let yourself relax completely. If you have time constraints, you may want to set an alarm in case you drift off.

7. After five to fifteen minutes of practicing the

Corpse Pose, slowly start to bring your awareness back into the room and into your body. Wiggle your fingers and toes a bit. When ready, come out of the pose with a deep inhalation as you gently roll to one side and bring yourself to seated position on the mat.

YOGA POSES FOR STAMINA

PLANK POSE (KUMBHAKASANA)

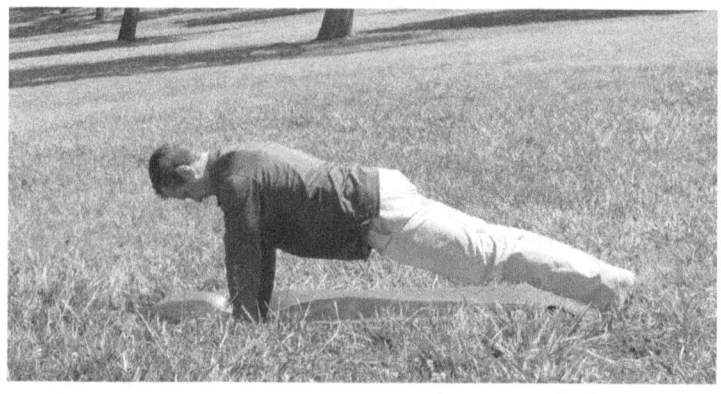

This is a key pose for increasing core strength and stability. In addition to increasing strength in your shoulders, legs, stomach, and back, you can stimulate your internal organs by pulling up on the perineum muscle, located on the floor of your pelvis. To make your body as "plank-like" as possible, keep pulling in your abdominal muscles while at the same time lowering your hips, and you'll see how challenging it can be to simply hold up your own body weight. By toning and firming up the muscles in your entire torso, you will automatically look thinner, even if your actual weight stays the same. Core muscles act like a natural girdle, and strengthening them helps improve posture as well as protects your back from injury.

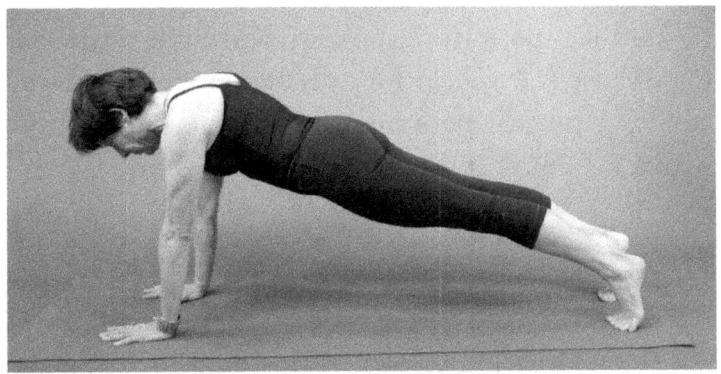

How to do it:

1. The pose looks like the top of a basic military-style push-up, except you do not go up and down. Instead, keep your body straight as a plank at the top of the push-up.

2. Start on your hands and knees, with your palms directly beneath your shoulders and your hips over your knees.

3. Extend your legs, keeping your toes tucked under. Straighten your arms, keeping your back straight and your body positioned—you guessed it—like a plank above the mat.

4. Rather than looking down toward your navel or forward, keep your gaze focused slightly ahead of

your hands, so that your neck stays in a straight line with your spine.

5. Hold for at least thirty seconds while breathing deeply through your nose.

UPWARD PLANK POSE (PURVOTTANASANA)

Another pose for core strengthening, Upward Plank Pose is excellent for opening up your chest and counteracting the poor posture that often comes from sitting for hours at the computer or driving.

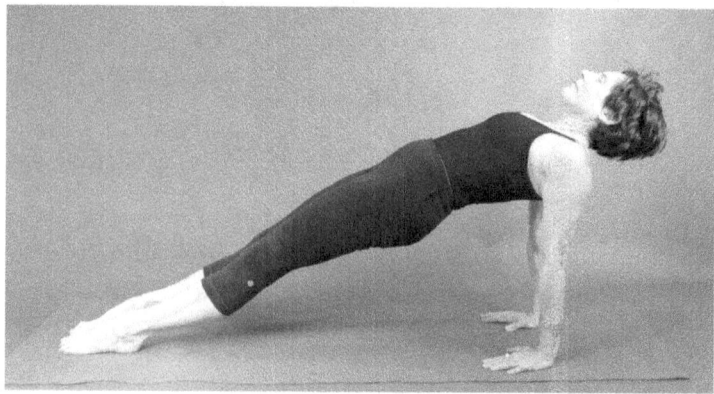

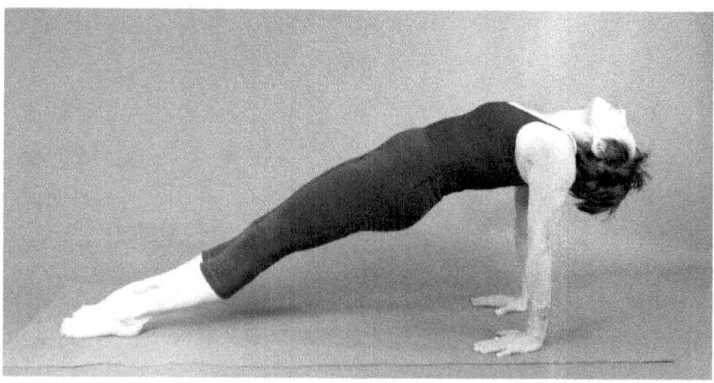

How to do it:

1. Sit on the floor with your hands several inches behind your hips and your fingers pointing forward. With your legs straight out in front of you, point your toes.

2. Lean back onto your hands, and, keeping your head in a straight line with your body, lift your hips up toward the ceiling. Press your shoulder blades against your back torso to support the lift of your chest.

3. Keeping your hips lifted, and (only if is comfortable) slowly drop your head back to look up at the ceiling, but do not overdo it by dropping your head back all the way down.

4. Hold for five breaths, then sit back down onto your mat. Try taking a forward bend as a counter stretch. Repeat one more time.

Variation: For more advanced pose, drop the head back, but do not attempt this if you have any neck injuries or if it's uncomfortable.

EAGLE POSE (GARUDASANA)

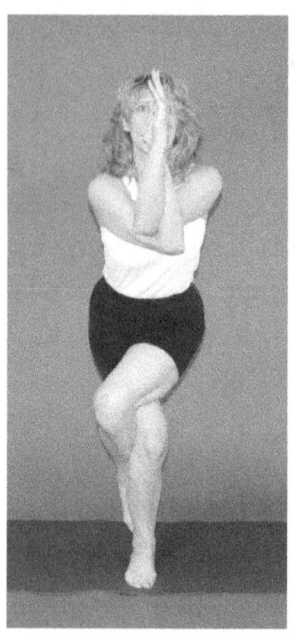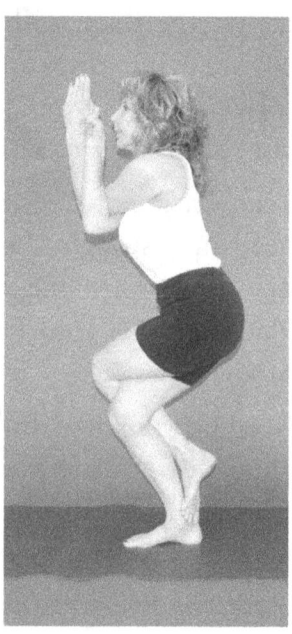

To be effective, every yoga pose requires focus and concentration, especially Eagle Pose. This stamina- and balance-building pose has you standing on one foot, with the other foot wrapped around the calf of the standing leg and your arms bent at the elbows and intertwined in front of you. Not only will this pose help you develop your concentration (or you won't be able to do it), but the posture loosens and stretches the muscles in the hips, upper back, and shoulders. This pose quickly relieves tension that develops from working at your desk all day.

How to do it:

1. Stand with your legs shoulder-width apart.

2. Exhale and extend your arms out to each side, parallel to the floor, as you widen your back. Inhale and cross your arms in front of you with the left arm above the right and bend your elbows. Ensure your left elbow is nestled in the crook of your right arm as you raise your forearms perpendicular to the floor. Inhale and place the backs of your hands together if possible; if not, grab your thumb.

3. After your elbows are hooked together, move your left hand to your left and your right hand to your right so the palms face each other. Inhale and press the palms together as closely as you can. Exhale and lift your elbows as you stretch your fingers toward the ceiling. Press your elbows down.

4. Inhale and bend your knees slightly. Shifting your weight, balance on your left foot, then lift your right leg up and cross your right thigh over your left thigh.

5. Point the toes of your right foot toward the floor, bring the foot back, and hook the top of it behind the lower portion of your left calf if you can. Inhale and concentrate on your balance. If you find that you cannot wrap your foot behind the calf, just touch your right toes to the ground on the outside of the standing left leg.

6. Continue to inhale and exhale as you hold the pose for as long as you can, at least fifteen seconds, and up to thirty seconds if possible. Unwind back to standing with an exhale and repeat on other side.

CRESCENT POSE (ANJANEYASANA)

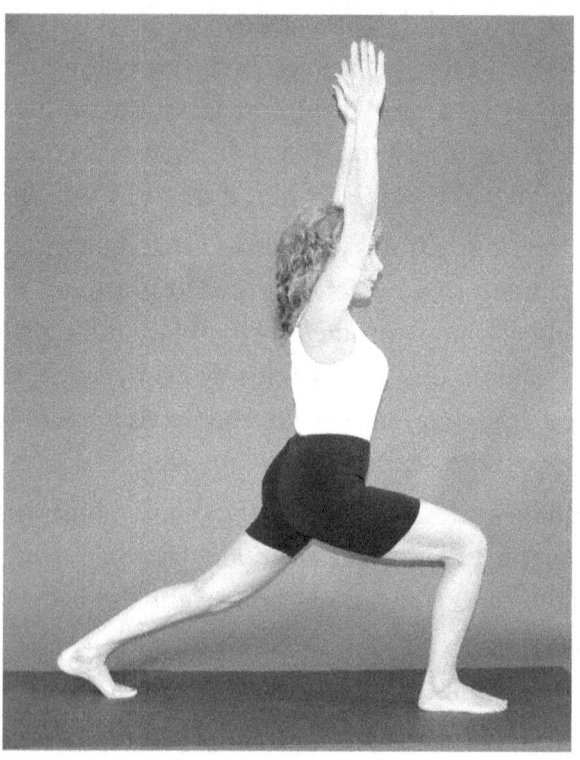

Variation 1 – Ball of the rear foot on the mat

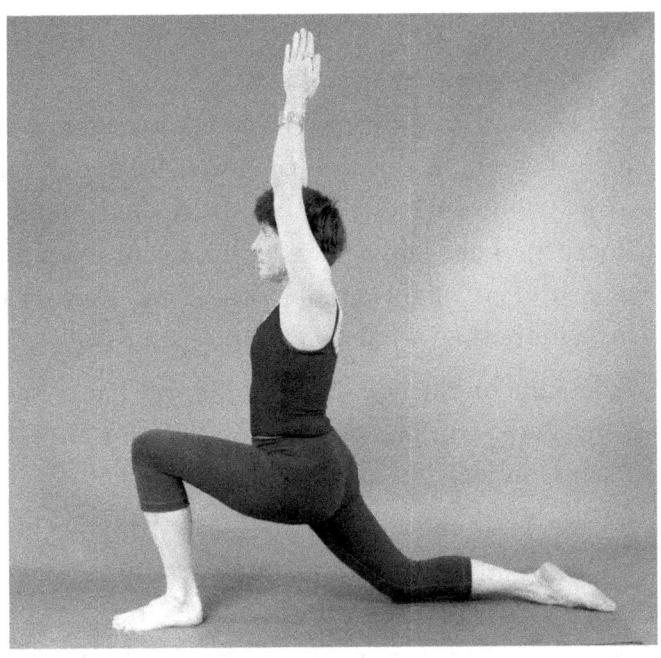

Variation 2 – Top of the rear foot and knee on the mat

Crescent Pose (or Crescent Lunge Pose) helps speed up your metabolism by working major muscle groups and increasing the heart rate. It burns calories like crazy. It's also good for strengthening the legs and opening up the groin area where the torso meets the legs. This area is significantly short and tight on almost everyone who sits most of the time at work. This pose works the large muscle groups in your thigh and hip areas as well as your gluteus, spinal erector, and latissimus back muscles.

How to do it:

1. Stand with your hands on your hips, step back with one leg, and keep the heel lifted with weight on the ball of the foot. Position the other leg far enough away from your body so that when you bend your knee, the knee stays over the foot, not extending past it. This might entail opening up your legs a little more than what you would expect.

2. Balancing on the ball of the foot in the back, lower your body straight down, not forward over the front bent leg.

3. Engage your abdominal muscles so that your body stays in a straight line, and don't let your abdomen bulge forward. Then lift your arms up toward the sky, trying to get your upper arms as close to your ears as you can.

4. You can point your fingers at the sky or clasp your hands with just the index fingers extended. Look straight ahead or look up if your neck feels comfortable doing this. This pose can also be modified and done with the back knee and top of the foot on the ground. (See Variation 2 photo, above.)

5. Stay in the posture for fifteen to thirty seconds, then release and change legs. Keep breathing.

CRESCENT POSE WITH SPINAL TWIST
(PARIVRTTA ANJANEYASANA)

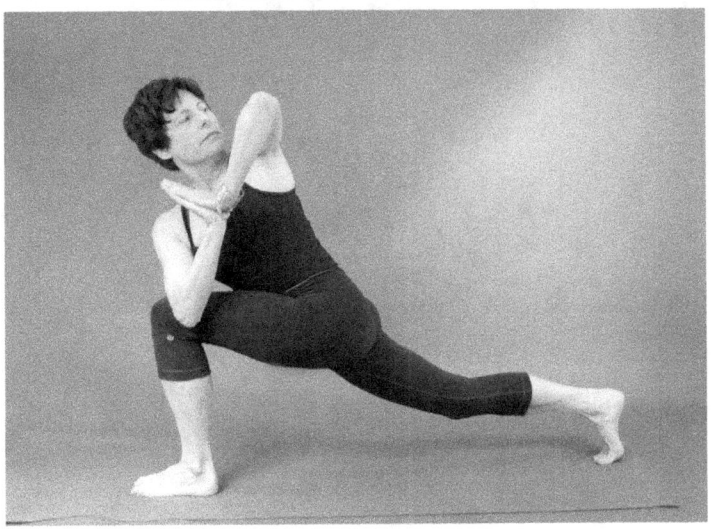

Crescent Pose with Spinal Twist (or Twisting Crescent Lunge) is a challenging variation on the previous pose, a strength and balance posture that works toward creating stability throughout the entire body, but especially the core. Twisting the torso applies pressure to your internal organs, toning them and increasing their ability to detoxify your body. After twisting, your torso and digestive organs are flushed with oxygen-rich blood, which helps remove toxins while improving digestion. This pose also stretches and tones the legs, hips, and buttocks, as well as opens the chest, shoulders, and arms. It improves balance and increases both energy and confidence.

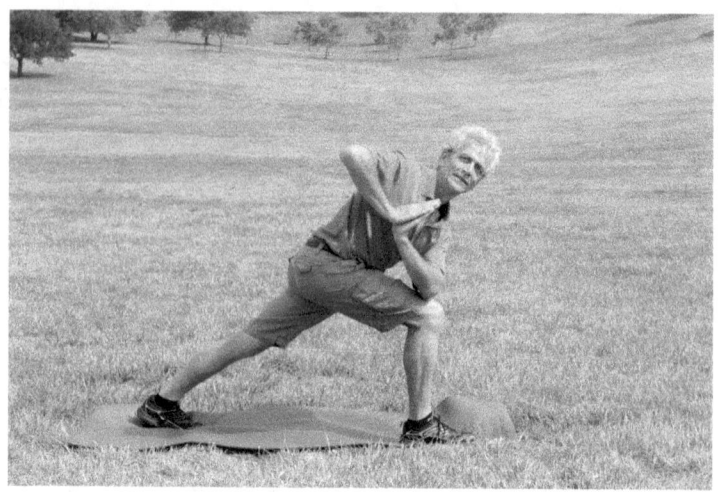

How to do it:

(Note: Until you get to Step 8, the pose is the same as Crescent Pose)

1. Begin in Downward Facing Dog. With an exhalation, step your right foot forward between your hands.

2. Bend your front knee to ninety degrees, aligning your knee directly over the heel of your front foot. Your feet should be hip-width apart with both feet facing forward, and your front shin should be perpendicular to the floor.

3. Come onto the ball of your back foot, lifting your heel and drawing it forward so it aligns directly over your back toes. Make sure your front shin stays vertical. Bring that foot forward as needed to

make sure that your knee does not move forward past your ankle, as this strains the knee.

4. Lift your back knee. Straighten your back leg completely. Keep the ball of your back foot firmly on the ground.

5. With your back leg strong and active, gently draw your left hip forward as you press your right hip back, squaring your hips so they are parallel to the top edge of your mat.

Beginner's Modification: If it is too difficult to keep your back knee raised, lower your knee to the floor and slide your entire leg back a few inches. Untuck your back toes and rest the top of your back foot on the floor.

6. Inhale as you raise your torso to an upright position, pointing your tailbone toward the earth and contracting the muscles in your abdomen so your stomach doesn't push forward. Sweep your arms overhead. Turn your arms so your palms face each other. Gently tilt your head and gaze up at a space between your thumbs.

7. Lower your arms and bring your palms together in prayer position at your chest. Bring your head back down so that your gaze is level with the horizon.

Now continue into Crescent Pose with Spinal Twist:

8. Exhaling, twist your torso to the right so that your left shoulder is pointing down toward your right

knee. Bring your left elbow to the outside of your right thigh.

9. Press your upper left arm against your thigh and turn your chest to the right.

10. Tuck your tailbone under and engage the muscles of your abdomen to help stabilize your core.

11. Extend and stretch up through the crown of your head, lengthening your upper body. Draw your shoulder blades down and firm them into your upper back.

12. Hold for up to one minute, breathing deeply. Exhaling, release your hands back to the mat and step back into Downward Dog. Repeat on the other side.

CHAIR POSE (UTKATASANA)

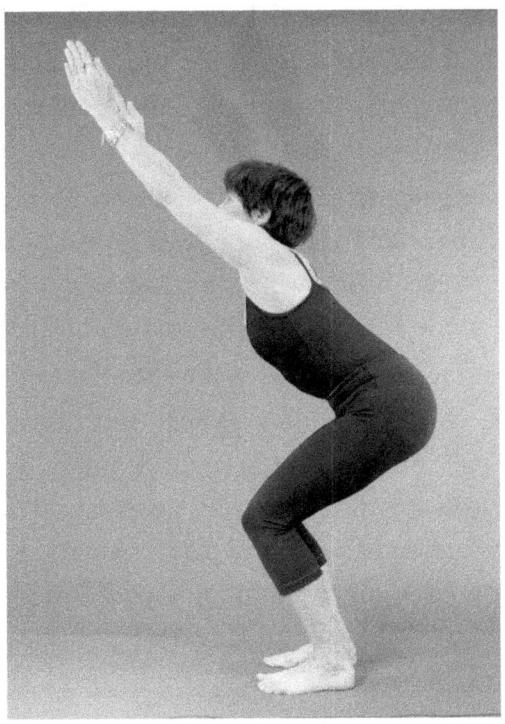

This pose is especially effective for weight loss because it engages 70 percent of all the muscles in your body, which includes the back, abdominals, glutes, and all the thigh muscles. It is excellent for raising your heart rate and increasing your metabolism.

In this pose, be sure that you're not hunching up your shoulders around your ears. It is easy to do, because it feels like you're getting more of a stretch, but try to remember to slide the shoulder blades down while you reach forward.

How to do it:

1. With your feet parallel to each other and slightly apart, raise your arms over your head with palms facing inward, or join the palms together. Keep your upper arms next to your ears. Take a breath.

2. Exhaling, bend your knees, trying to make your thighs parallel to the floor. In this pose, your knees will project out over your feet. Try to make a right angle between your upper and lower leg and between your thighs and your body.

3. Move your shoulders down and back, engage your abdominal muscles, and point your tailbone toward the floor. Stay in this pose for thirty seconds, breathing as much as necessary. Keep your breathing deep, even though your breaths might come faster. Release on an exhale and stand up.

DOWNWARD FACING DOG
(ADHO MUKHA SVANASANA)

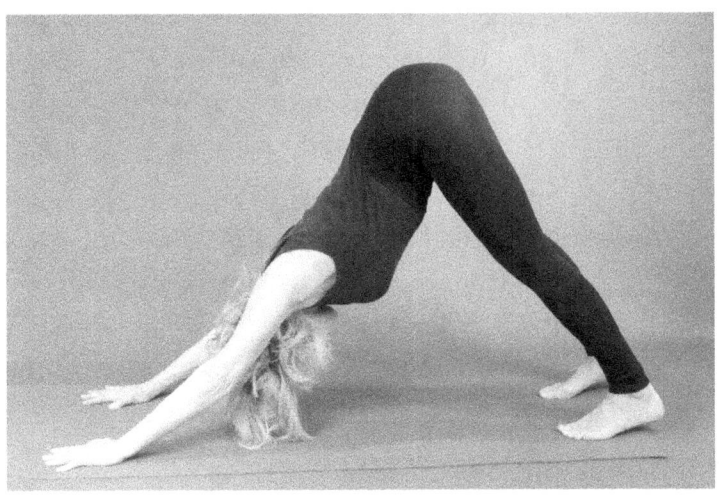

Downward Facing Dog pose stretches and engages the stomach, shoulders, back, arms, and legs. It reverses gravity for your entire upper body and takes pressure off the heart, which makes it less work to get blood flowing to the organs in the upper body and the brain. Like other inversion poses, the reverse action of gravity on the body gets the lymphatic fluid flowing in opposite directions, which helps remove toxins from your system. This pose is also good for metabolic balance and elimination because it relieves gravitational pressure on the abdomen.

How to do it:

1. Start on the floor on your hands and knees. Make sure your knees are directly below your hips and your hands are slightly forward of your shoulders. Spread your palms with your middle fingers pointing straight ahead and tuck your toes under.

2. Exhale and lift your knees away from the floor. At first, keep the knees slightly bent and the heels lifted away from the floor. Lengthen your tailbone away from the back of your pelvis and press it lightly toward the floor. Lift your hips toward the sky. Inhale.

3. Then, with an exhalation, push your top thighs back and stretch your heels down toward the floor. Straighten your knees, but be sure not to lock them.

4. Engage the outer arms and press the bases of the index fingers actively into the floor. Slide your shoulder blades down your back. Keep the head between the upper arms; don't let it hang.

5. Stay in the pose anywhere from thirty seconds to three minutes.

6. To come out of the pose, drop your knees to the mat, untuck your toes, and rest in Child's Pose until your blood pressure normalizes, then sit up.

Downward Facing Dog is one of the poses in the traditional Sun Salutation sequence. It's also an excellent yoga asana all on its own.

UPWARD FACING DOG
(URDHVA MUKHA SVANASANA)

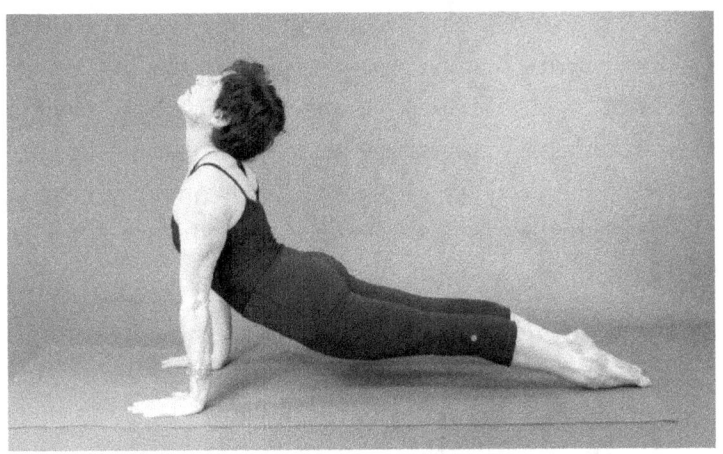

Upward Facing Dog is a simple pose designed to strengthen the legs and buttocks, as well as the shoulders, torso, arms and wrists. This pose also stretches out the shoulders and back and opens the chest and stomach. The pose is being introduced here, as it will be used later as part of the Sun Salutation sequence.

How to do it:

1. Lie flat on your belly. Stretch your body along the floor. Stretch your arms down the length of your body and relax.

2. Bend your arms and rest your palms on the floor on either side of your chest. Your legs should still be lying flat on the floor with the tops of the feet on your mat. Look straight ahead of you with your

chin resting on the mat.

3. Inhale and squeeze your shoulder blades together.

4. Exhale and press your hands down. Straighten your arms, bringing your torso and legs up off the floor as if you were doing push-up. Your weight should be distributed between your hands and toes. All your weight rests on the tops of your feet and your palms, with your body bowing downward in between like a hammock.

5. Lengthen the sides of your body and keep your neck long. Draw your shoulder blades deeply back to lift your heart forward and up. Hold the pose for three to five breaths, then release your body back towards the floor and lie on your stomach or pike back up to Downward Facing Dog for several breaths before resting.

We will revisit this pose later as part of the Sun Salutation.

STANDING SPLITS
(URDHVA PRASARITS EKA PADASANA)

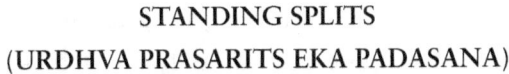

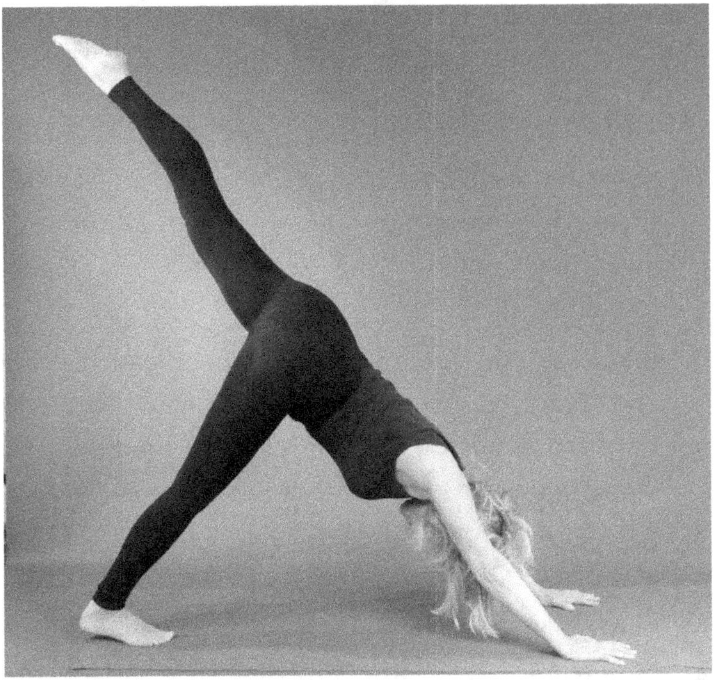

Standing Splits stretches the whole back side of the body, particularly the hamstrings and calves. It strengthens the thighs, knees, and ankles, and also stretches the groin muscles, aiding in lymphatic drainage. This is considered a stamina and balance pose because supporting your body's weight on one leg while upside down will greatly challenge and improve your balance.

Since your heart is above your head in this pose, it includes all the benefits of an inversion, including relief from headaches, anxiety, fatigue, insomnia, and mild depression. The increased flow of blood to the brain calms your nervous system and helps to improve memory and concentration and relieve stress.

How to do it:

1. Standing with your arms at your sides, let your breath become steady and rhythmic. Draw your awareness inward and focus on the present moment.

2. Inhale as you reach your arms overhead. Exhale and bend at the hips, coming into Standing Forward Bend. Bring both hands to the floor and straighten your legs, without locking your knees.

3. Beginners Modification: If your hands don't rest easily on the floor, place each hand on a yoga block, or low chair seat.

4. Shift your weight onto your right foot and equally across both hands. Then, raise your left leg up as high as you can. Try not to open your hips to the left as you do this; simply lift the leg behind you with the back of the leg toward the ceiling.

5. Internally rotate your left thigh (rotate your left hip down slightly) and square your hips toward the floor (doing so may require you to lower your left leg a bit).

6. If you need a little more challenge, walk your hands back (in the direction of your standing

foot) to deepen the stretch and bring your torso closer to your right leg. Breathe deeply and relax your shoulders. Tuck your chin into your chest; don't crunch or compress the back of your neck. Keep the knee and foot of your standing leg facing directly forward.

7. Hold for five breaths. Then slowly lower your left leg to the floor, coming back into Standing Forward Bend. Repeat the pose on the other side for the same amount of time.

Standing Split is a powerful stretch when practiced correctly. If your hamstrings are tight, this pose may seem impossible to ever achieve! But with practice and patience, your hamstrings will become more flexible. Remember to take it slowly and never force the pose.

TRIANGLE POSE (UTTHITA TRIKONASANA)

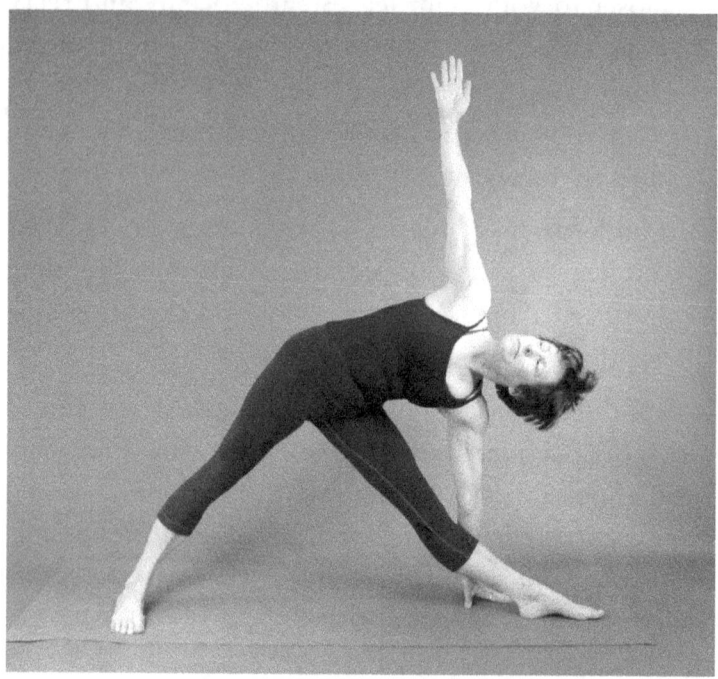

This pose is a real multitasker—a deep stretch for the hamstrings, groins, and hips. Triangle Pose also opens the chest and shoulders. It helps relieve stress, lower back pain, and sluggish digestion. This pose strengthens and tones the muscles in the waist, arms, shoulders, thighs, hips, and back. It also stimulates the internal organs and flushes the kidneys, improving removal of metabolic waste. Triangle improves overall balance and stability, both physically and mentally, increasing confidence and balance, creating poise and grace both on and off the mat.

How to do it:

1. Begin by standing sideways at the top of your mat with your feet hip distance apart and your arms at your sides. Pay attention to your breath, making your breath soft and full. Take a moment to tune into your body and draw your awareness inward.

2. Step your feet wide apart, about four to five feet. Check to ensure that your heels are aligned with each other.

3. Turn your right foot out ninety degrees so your toes are pointing to the top of the mat. The center of your right kneecap should be aligned with the center of your right ankle. Pivot your left foot slightly inward. Your back toes should be at a forty-five-degree angle, with the heel pointing toward the back corner of your mat.

4. Raise your arms to the side to shoulder height so they're parallel to the floor. Your arms should be aligned directly over your legs. With your palms facing down, reach actively from fingertip to fingertip. Notice if you are contracting or lifting your shoulders, and press your shoulders down slightly.

5. On an exhale, stretch out your body to the right and reach your right hand a few inches in the same direction as your right foot is pointed. Move your left hip to the left so your hips shift in the opposite direction from the way your right arm is reaching. Begin to pivot your upper body down, folding at

your right hip. Keep your right ear, shoulder, and knee on the same plane—do not let your torso drop forward. Turn your left palm forward with your fingertips reaching toward the sky.

6. Rest your right hand wherever it lands on your outer shin or ankle. If you are more flexible, slide your hand down and place your right fingertips or palm on the floor to the outside of your right shin. You can also place your hand on a block. Align your shoulders so your left shoulder is directly above your right shoulder.

7. Gently turn your head down to gaze at your right thumb (as long as this does not cause any discomfort). Alternatively, you can look up at your raised hand, but this requires more balance. If turning your head at all is uncomfortable, simply keep your gaze straight ahead on the horizon.

8. Push down through the outer edge of your back foot. Extend equally through both sides of your waist, making sure your ribs are not humping up. Lengthen your spine, and keep your left arm in line with your shoulders.

9. Hold for up to one minute. To release, inhale and press firmly through your left heel as you lift your torso. Place your hands on your hips, turn to the left, reversing the position of your feet, extend your arms again, and repeat for the same length of time on that side.

REVOLVED TRIANGLE POSE
(PARIVRTTA TRIKONASANA)

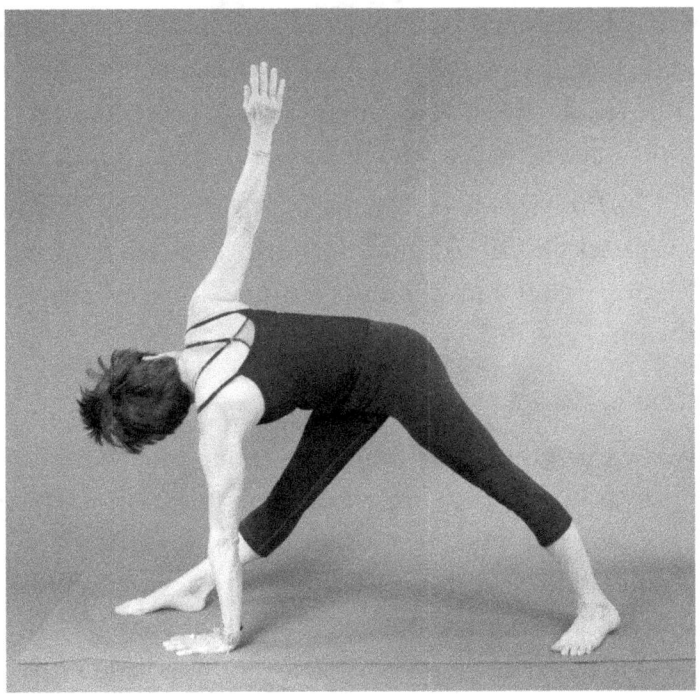

Revolved Triangle Pose is a standing, deep-twisting yoga pose that stretches the whole body. It squeezes and massages your digestive organs, while challenging your balance and concentration. Adding a twist to the torso massages your internal organs, which tones them and increases their ability to detoxify your body. Cleansing and toning these internal organs also improves metabolism, and is therapeutic for digestive troubles, including constipation. This pose also helps to relieve low back pain and sciatica due to the strengthening of the thigh, hip, and back muscles.

Twisted Triangle can be a great way to add detoxifying benefits to your practice and at the same time challenge your grace and balance. Practicing this pose on a regular basis will enhance your poise and focus while squeezing out toxins that can weigh you down.

Caution: If you are pregnant, avoid this pose. Those with neck injuries should not turn their heads to face the top hand but should continue looking straight ahead.

How to do it:

1. Begin standing at the top of your mat with your feet hip-distance apart and your arms at your sides. Step your feet about two to three feet apart and align your heels. (If you are transitioning from regular Triangle Pose to Revolved Triangle Pose, remember to step your back foot in a little bit.)

2. Turn your right foot out ninety degrees so your toes are pointing to the top of the mat. The center of your right kneecap should be aligned with the center of your right ankle. Pivot your left foot inward to a forty-five-degree angle.

3. Bring your hands to your hips and square your hips forward.

4. Reach with your left arm toward the ceiling, with your bicep next to your left ear. Reach up strongly through your left hand.

5. On an exhale, hinge forward from your hips, keeping your spine long. Reach forward to the front with your left hand, feeling the stretch all the way from your left hip to your left fingertips. Then place your left hand to the outside of your right foot (or on a yoga block that you've put there) as you open your torso to the right.

6. Use your right hand to draw your right hip back so it stays in line with your left hip.

7. Inhale and lengthen your spine again. Then exhale as you roll your right shoulder back and extend your right arm straight up toward the ceiling. Reach strongly through your right fingertips.

8. Turn your head to gaze at your right thumb.

9. Keep your hips level. Press down firmly through your back heel.

10. Hold the pose for up to one minute. To come out of the pose, gently release the twist. Then press firmly through your left heel. With an inhalation, lift your torso upright and lower your arms. Place your hands on your hips, turn to the left, reversing the position of your feet, and repeat for the same length of time on the opposite side.

Revolved Triangle Pose will work every muscle in your body when practiced correctly! You might want to experiment with these variations to find a version of the pose that works best for you right now. If you feel unsteady in the pose, there are a few modifications you can try to make the pose more suitable to your needs:

- Rest your back heel against a wall.

- A narrower stance will also be more stable, so step your back foot in slightly if you need extra support.

- Rest your bottom hand on a block.

- Beginners and those who are less flexible can rest the bottom hand near the inside of the front foot or on the shin of the front leg.

For more leverage to help roll your torso open, lift your back heel slightly. This will make the pose unstable, but you can press your back heel onto a folded yoga mat or against a wall for better balance.

Things to remember:

- Practicing Revolved Triangle will lengthen and stretch the whole body, rejuvenating your energy quickly.

- Keep your pelvis neutral and turn your trunk instead. Think of your hips as the anchor of this pose.

- Before coming into the twist, place your hands on your hip bones to determine whether your hips are squared to the front of your mat. Draw the hip of your front leg back and the opposite hip forward.

- Lift your belly in and up.

- Keep a straight line through your spine—do not let your spine round in the pose.

- Never force the twist! Only turn as far as it feels healthy and comfortable, then gently deepen the pose from there.

WARRIOR POSE I (VIRABHADRASANA I)

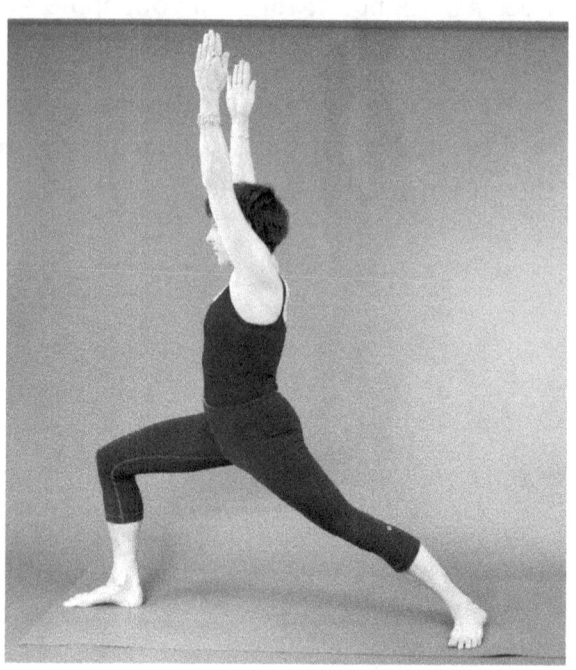

Warrior I is a standing yoga pose named after a mythological Hindu warrior, *Virabhadra*. An incarnation of the god Shiva, Virabhadra was fierce and powerful, with a thousand arms and hair and eyes of fire. Warrior I transforms the intensity of this deity into a pose that builds focus, power, and stability.

Warrior Pose I develops stamina, balance, and coordination, as well as stretches the whole front side of the body while strengthening the thighs, shoulders, and back. This pose opens up the chest and lungs, improving breathing capacity and invigorating the entire body. It encourages greater flexibility, strength, and range of motion in the feet, increasing circulation as it warms all of the muscles.

Beyond the physical posture, Warrior Pose I creates deep concentration. Focusing on your foundation and building the pose from the ground up reduces distractions and focuses your energy. Your mind becomes honed, calm, and clear.

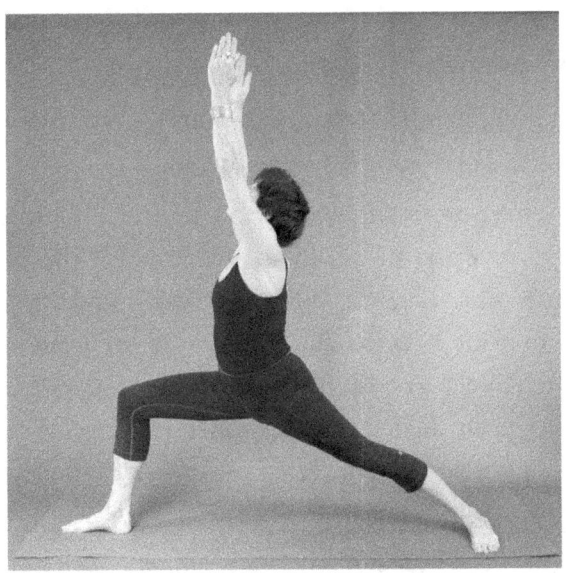

Caution: Those with neck injuries should keep their heads in a neutral position—do not look up at your hands (see photo on left, above). Anyone with a shoulder injury should keep his or her raised arms parallel to each other or slightly wider and be cautions to not stretch too far back.

How to do it:

1. Begin by standing with your feet hip-distance apart
    and your arms at your sides. Let your thoughts
    settle and focus on the present moment. Breathe
    deeply and evenly, calming your mind. Draw your
    awareness inward.

2. Exhale as you step your feet wide apart, about
    four to five feet.

3. Turn your right foot out ninety degrees so your
    toes are pointing to the top of the mat.

4. Pivot your left foot inward at a forty-five-degree
    angle. Turn your body to the right.

5. Align your front heel with the arch of your back
    foot. Keep your pelvis turned toward the front of
    your mat. If your hips are very tight, step your
    front foot toward the outer edge of your mat so
    your heels are aligned (instead of heel-to-arch).
    Step your feet as wide apart as necessary. This
    will give you more room to square the hips as you
    work on gaining flexibility.

6. Press your weight through your left heel. Then
    exhale as you bend your right knee over your right
    ankle. Your shin should be perpendicular to the
    floor. If your right knee extends beyond your right
    ankle, step your left foot back farther.

7. Be aware of your back (left) foot, and press the
    outside of the foot into the mat. Be sure your

weight is distributed evenly on both feet.

8. Reach up strongly through your arms. Broaden across the front of the torso, lengthen the sides of your waist, and lift through your chest. Keep your palms and fingers active and reaching, but press your shoulders down. If your shoulders are tight, keep your arms shoulder-distance apart or wider; they should not be lifted around your ears.

9. You can keep your arms parallel or press your palms together. Place your hands on your hips if you have a shoulder injury or if you're using this pose to build strength and flexibility in your lower body.

10. Gently tilt your head back and gaze up at your thumbs. Keep your shoulders dropped away from your ears. Feel your shoulder blades pressing firmly inward.

11. Press down through the outer edge of your back foot, keeping your back leg straight.

12. Hold for up to one minute, breathing deeply.

13. To release the pose, press your weight through your back heel and straighten your front leg. Lower your arms. Turn to the left, reversing the position of your feet, and repeat for the same length of time on the opposite side.

If you're looking to deepen the pose or lighten the level of exertion, there are simple modifications you can make. Try these changes to find a version of the pose that works best for you right now:

- If your hips are very tight, step your feet as wide apart as necessary. This will give you more room to square the hips as you work on gaining flexibility.

- If your shoulders are tight, keep your arms shoulder-distance apart or wider when they are raised.

- Place your hands on your hips if you have a shoulder injury or if you're using this pose to build strength and flexibility in your lower body.

Warrior I requires focus on various points of alignment. There is a lot to remember to execute the pose correctly, so keep the following information in mind when practicing:

- Build the pose from the ground up. Work on getting the foot and leg placement first. Orient your feet, then adjust your legs. Finally, align your hips.

- Place your hands on your hip bones to determine whether they are squared to the front of your mat. Draw the hip of your front leg back and the opposite hip forward.

- Lengthen your tailbone toward the floor, rather than dipping your pelvis forward. This allows for greater length in your lower back.

- Press back firmly with the top of your back thigh before bending your front knee. This helps to stabilize and root down through the outer edge of your back foot. Keep that stabilization as you bend the front knee.

- Keep your weight even across the three points of both feet: the center of your heel, the ball of your big toe, and the ball of your baby toe. This will help keep your arches actively lifting.

Warrior I can be a powerful way to build concentration, balance, and focus. It creates strength in all areas of life—physical, mental, emotional, and spiritual. Practicing this pose regularly will help you to face the challenges of daily life with equanimity and poise.

WARRIOR POSE II (VIRABHADRASANA II)

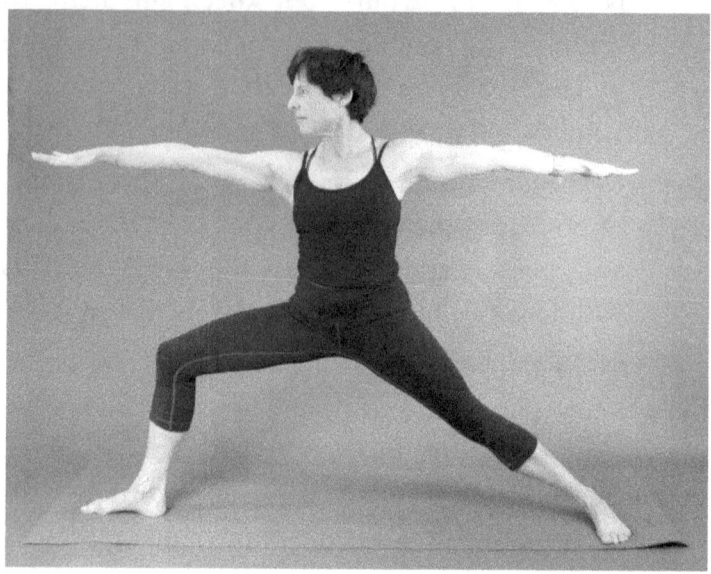

This is a standing pose that enhances strength, stability, and concentration; creates a powerful stretch for the legs, groins, and chest; and also increases stamina. More than just a physical posture, Warrior Pose II increases your ability to concentrate. As you hone your gaze, you direct your mind clearly and with intention. Distractions disappear and your energy becomes powerful and focused. It also encourages good posture, helps to relieve backaches, and stimulates healthy digestion.

How to do it:

1. Begin in Mountain Pose, standing with your feet hip-distance apart and your arms at your sides.

Let go of distractions. Notice the quality of your breath. Draw your awareness inward.

2. Exhale as you step your feet wide apart, about four to five feet. Check to ensure that your heels are aligned with each other.

3. Turn your right foot out ninety degrees so your toes are pointing to the top of the mat. Pivot your left foot slightly inward. Your back toes should be at a forty-five-degree angle.

4. Lift through the arches of your feet while rooting down through your ankles.

5. Raise your arms to the side to shoulder height, so they're parallel to the floor. Your arms should be aligned directly over your legs. With your palms facing down, reach actively from fingertip to fingertip.

6. On an exhale, bend your front knee. Align your knee directly over the ankle of your front foot. Your front shin should be perpendicular to the floor. Sink your hips low, eventually bringing your front thigh parallel to the floor. Make sure your front shin stays vertical. Widen your stance as needed to make sure that your knee does not move forward past your ankle.

7. Press down through the outer edge of your back foot and keep your back leg straight.

8. Keep your torso perpendicular to the floor, with your head directly over your tailbone. Do not lean

toward your front leg.

9. Turn your head to gaze out across the tip of your right middle finger. Broaden across your collarbones and lengthen the space between your shoulder blades. Stretch your arms in opposite directions, engaging your triceps. Drop your shoulders and lift your chest.

10. Draw your belly in toward your spine. Keep your torso open to the side, not turned toward the front leg.

11. Hold for up to one minute.

12. To release, inhale as you press down through your back foot and straighten your front leg. Lower your arms. Turn to the left, reversing the position of your feet, and repeat for the same length of time on the opposite side.

BOW POSE (DHANURASANA)

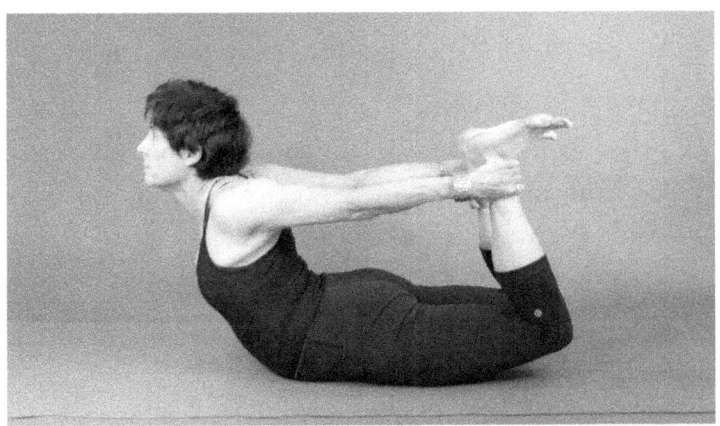

Bow Pose, which is a prone back bend, boosts energy and keeps your metabolism high. It strengthens your back muscles while stretching and opening up the front of your body. It also opens up the heart area significantly, and by opening up the intercostal muscles in the rib cage, the bow pose trains your breathing muscles to function more efficiently with less effort.

How to do it:

1. Lying face down on your mat, bend your legs at the knee and flex your feet at the ankle. Reaching your arms straight back, grab your ankle or shin with the palms facing either in or out (whatever feels best to you is what works).

2. Press your legs back to arch and lift your upper body, and then reach up toward the ceiling with your feet.

3. Take five deep inhales and exhales and feel your diaphragm muscle working. As you expand it, you might even be able to rock your body with your breath a little.

4. After coming out of the pose (gracefully), rest on your stomach with your head resting on your folded arms facing to the right to relieve any tension in the neck that the pose might have generated. Repeat the pose and rest for another thirty seconds with your head facing to the left.

BRIDGE POSE (SETU BANDHA SARVANGASANA)

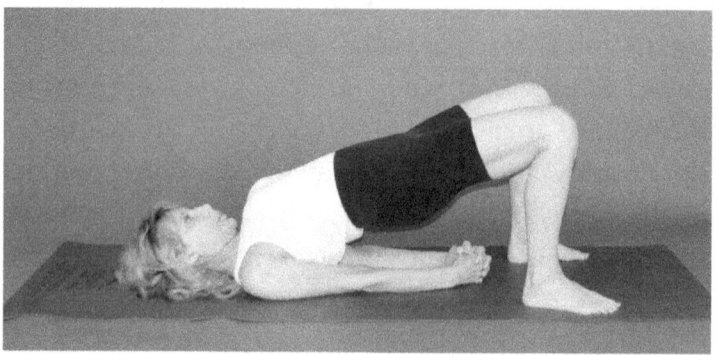

The Bridge Pose, like the plow, is a gentle but powerful inversion that works with gravity to reverse the flow of blood to the heart and brain, increase lymph flow and open the chest and shoulder area. As the hips rise, the chest is pressed up toward the chin and the movement massages the thyroid gland. As mentioned earlier, stimulating the thyroid encourages production of the hormones that regulate the body's metabolism.

This pose engages the hamstrings, large muscles of the back of the thigh, and elevates the heart rate if held for thirty seconds or more. Aim for a fifteen-second hold to start, then gradually increase.

Beginner's modification: If the front of your shoulders are too tight to work your arms underneath your body, keep your arms on the floor at your sides.

How to do it:

1. Lie on your back with your knees bent and your heels fairly close to your hips. You will notice, if you have any difficulty lifting your hips, that you get the best leverage if your heels are directly under your knees.

2. Keep your arms flat on the mat by your side for the first part of the pose.

3. Press your hips up toward the sky, attempting to make a straight "plank" from your knees to your shoulders, using your hamstring muscles and not your buttocks. Try to relax your butt and avoid squeezing.

4. If you can rock yourself from side to side and lift your body up enough to bring your upper arms behind your back and clasp your hands, this completes the pose. If you can't do that for now, allow your arms to stay at your sides, and you will still gain significant benefit.

In addition to massaging the thyroid gland, this

pose engages the perineum muscle, which in turn stimulates either the testes (if you're male) or the ovaries (for females). The perineum muscle is the muscle at the base of the body located between the anal sphincter and the urogenital muscles. With practice, this muscle can be isolated and engaged for a variety of purposes—when you practice contracting this muscle, you are strengthening your pelvic floor muscles. A strong pelvic floor can help prevent urinary incontinence later in life. For men, exercising the perineal muscles can prevent possible prostate problems and impotence. Women can perform perineal exercises to prepare for and recover from childbirth as well as prevent uterine prolapse.

YOGA POSES FOR BALANCE

MOUNTAIN POSE (TADASANA)

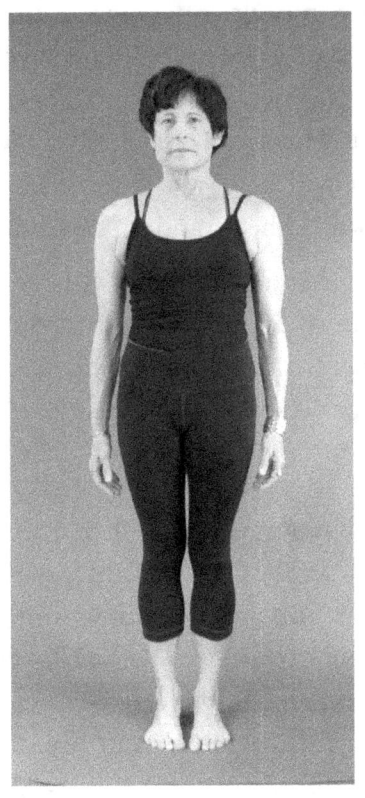

It might look like you're just standing there, but Mountain Pose is an active pose that helps improve posture, balance, and serenity. This pose steadies the mind and body, rewarding you with the ability to face life with a calm focus. Practicing the pose with steady and smooth breathing will help relieve stress and improve concentration.

Mountain Pose is the foundational pose for all standing yoga postures—this is the pose from which every other standing pose in your practice is born. The alignment, muscle movements, and mindset you learn in Mountain Pose are applied every time you do a standing yoga pose, so it's important to learn how to do it correctly. Once you understand the proper form of the pose, it will be easier to gain and maintain the alignment for all other standing poses and inversions.

A correctly executed Mountain Pose will use every muscle in the body. It improves posture and strengthens the thighs, knees, ankles, abdomen, and buttocks. It is also helpful for relieving sciatica.

How to do it:

1. Stand with your feet together and your arms at your sides. Press your weight evenly across each entire foot. Breathe steadily and rhythmically. Draw your awareness inward. Focus on the present moment, letting all worries and concerns fade away. Just focus on your breath.

2. Press your big toes together (separate your heels slightly). Lift your toes and spread them apart. Then place them back down on the mat. If you have trouble balancing, stand with your feet six inches apart (or wider).

3. Press down through your heels and straighten your legs, keeping just a slight microbend in your

knees, and avoid locking them. Ground your feet firmly into the earth, pressing evenly across all four corners of both feet.

4. Draw the top of your thighs up and back, engaging the quadriceps. Rotate your thighs slightly inward, widening your sit bones.

5. Tuck in your tailbone slightly, but don't round your lower back. Lift the back of your thighs, but don't squeeze your buttocks.

6. Bring your pelvis to its neutral position. Do not let your front hip bones point down or up; instead, point them straight forward. Draw your belly in slightly.

7. As you inhale, elongate through your torso. Elongate your neck. Exhale and release your shoulder blades away from your head, toward the back of your waist.

8. Broaden across your collarbones, keeping your shoulders in line with the sides of your body. Press your shoulder blades toward the back ribs, but don't squeeze them together. Keep your arms straight, fingers extended, and triceps firm. Allow your inner arms to rotate slightly outward.

9. Your ears, shoulders, hips, and ankles should all be in one line (if you could see yourself from the side, your posture would be gorgeous!).

10. Keep your breathing smooth and even. With each

exhalation, feel your spine elongating. Softly gaze forward toward the horizon line. Hold the pose for up to one minute.

This pose will help you to be more aware in general of your posture, even when standing in line at the grocery store. And what situation can you think of that won't benefit from you dropping your shoulders and taking a deep breath?

SHOULDERSTAND (SARVANGASANA)

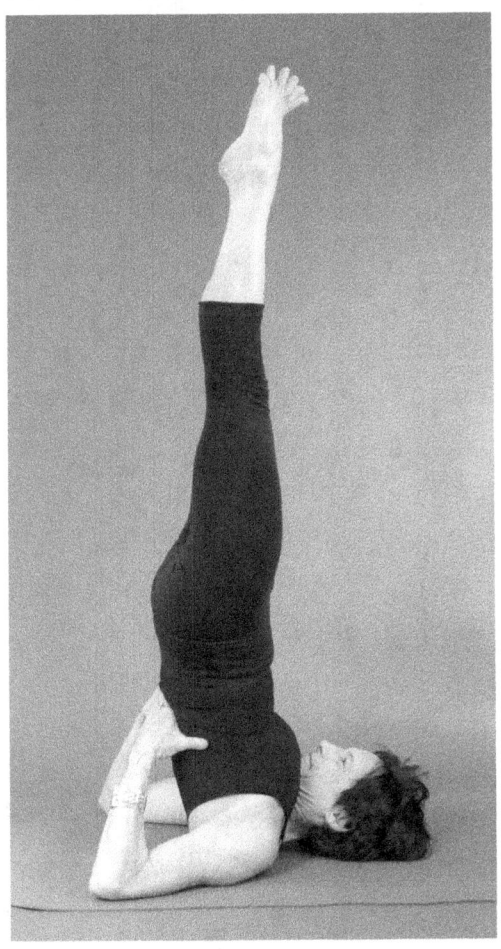

One of the best poses for toning up the body for weight loss, Shoulderstand is often referred to as the "queen" of all yoga postures, with Headstand being deemed the "king." The many benefits of Shoulderstand cannot be understated, as it is a complete pose, meaning that it aides in the function of the entire body.

Some of the positive effects of Shoulderstand include:

- Stimulates the endocrine system and balances the thyroid and hypothalamus glands, allowing for proper hormone function.

- Strengthens the heart and respiratory system by placing the body in an inverted position. Shoulderstand reduces strain on the heart. Brings more blood to the brain via gravity.

- Has a soothing effect on the parasympathetic nervous system.

- The change in gravitational pull on the body affects the abdominal organs so that the bowels move freely and constipation is relieved.

- Increases strength and flexibility by strengthening the upper body, legs, and abdomen. The posture opens the upper chest and stretches the neck and shoulders; strong back and gluteus muscles are needed to stay in the pose.

- Better complexion. Due to increased blood flow to the face, yoga practitioners notice an improved complexion with a consistent Shoulderstand practice.

- Done before bedtime, Shoulderstand can promote deeper sleep.

Caution: Shoulderstand has the potential for over-stretching the muscles and tendons in the neck, so care should be exercised in setting up for and staying in the posture. When practicing Shoulderstand for the first time, fold up a blanket and place it under your shoulders, so that it comes below your seventh cervical vertebrae, while your neck and head remain on the mat. This additional height for the body takes some pressure off the back of the neck and reduces the angle at which the neck gets stretched.

You might feel awkward getting into the pose for the first time. Take your time and keep your mind on your alignment. Once you're in the pose, you will gain all of the benefits.

How to do it:

1. Begin by lying flat on your back with your legs extended and your arms at your sides, palms down. Bend your knees and place the soles of your feet flat on the floor.

2. On an inhale, use your abdominal muscles to lift your legs and hips off the floor. Curl your torso and bring your knees in toward your face. Then lift your hips and bring your torso perpendicular to the floor.

3. Bend your elbows and place your hands on your lower back with your fingertips pointing up toward the ceiling. Keep your elbows on the

ground, shoulder-width apart. Do not let your elbows splay out to the sides.

4. When you are comfortable, lift your thighs so they are vertical to the floor, keeping your knees bent. Draw your tailbone toward your pubic bone. Then straighten your legs fully and reach your feet up to the ceiling. Lift through the balls of your feet.

5. Try to bring your shoulders, hips, and feet into one line. This is most easily accomplished by pushing the hips forward (toward your head) and the feet back.

6. Bring your big toes together, and slightly rotate your legs inward. Spread out your toes.

7. Keep your head and neck in line with your spine and do not turn your head. Draw your shoulder blades firmly into your upper back. Keep a space between your chin and chest, and soften your throat. Gaze toward your chest.

8. Hold the pose for one to three minutes; more advanced practitioners can hold the pose for five minutes or longer. To release the pose, slowly lower your feet back to the ground, coming into Plow Pose with your hands supporting your back. Then, release your hands to your sides and slowly roll down, one vertebra at a time, bending your knees if you need to.

As with all inversions, Shoulderstand will invigorate

and rejuvenate your whole body when practiced correctly. It's important that you perform the pose with correct alignment; otherwise, it's possible to injure your neck. Be sure to take it slowly and make whatever adjustments you need to reduce discomfort. Keep the following information in mind when practicing this pose:

- Lift your chest to your chin instead of bringing your chin toward your chest.

- Never turn your head in Shoulderstand; protect your neck.

- It can be difficult to gauge how vertical your legs are in the pose, so ask someone to assess your pose.

- Breathe consciously throughout the pose. Continually bringing your awareness back to your breath will help relax your mind and body even further.

- Take the pose slowly—do not swing your legs up. Keep your legs active and firm with straight knees and do not squeeze your buttocks. Keep lifting through your feet; that will engage the legs without squeezing the buttocks.

Take your time coming out of the pose. You can drop your legs down into Plow Pose before gently lowering your hips. Some people like to do this pose as the last one in their practice before relaxing in Corpse

Pose. In any case, rest for a minute before standing up. You may feel slightly dizzy if you release the pose and stand up too quickly.

Be patient. With time and practice, you will gain the strength and poise needed to hold the pose for several minutes.

TREE POSE (VRKSASANA)

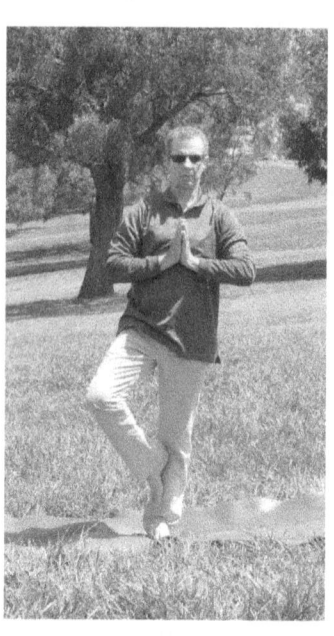 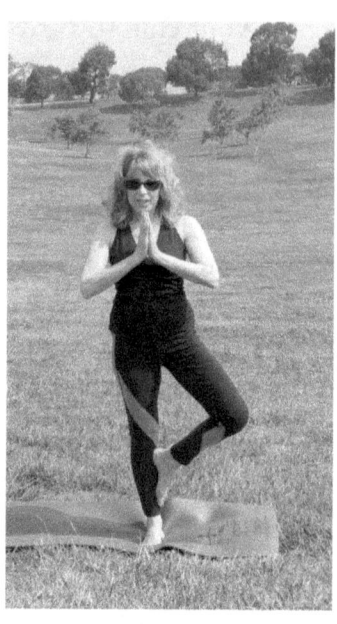

By regularly practicing balancing poses, you gain concentration, focus, poise, and coordination—and a steady and balanced mind. Tree Pose connects you to the earth, as you root down through your standing foot. As you balance in the pose, feel the slight and gentle sway of your body. Just like a tree in the breeze, you'll grow in confidence, standing tall as you face life's challenges with grace and ease.

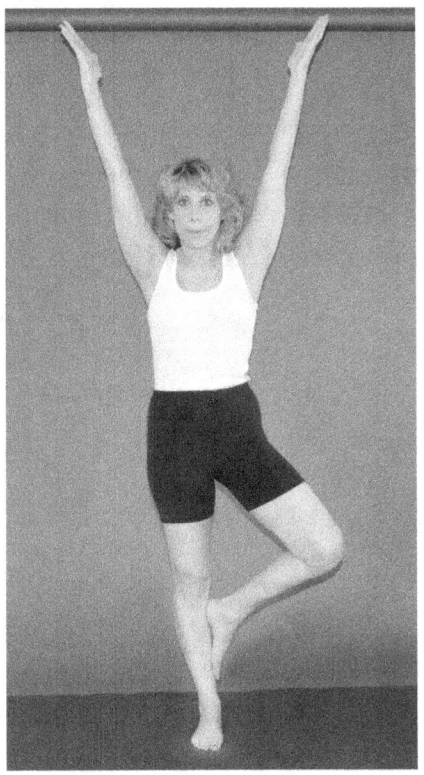

Practicing balancing poses in yoga, such as Tree Pose, will help you gain both physical *and* mental steadiness and poise. It will improve your focus and concentration while calming your mind.

Tree Pose, with its calming and meditative benefits, is like a standing variation of a seated meditation posture. Keeping calm and focused while balancing on one foot will teach you to sway gently like a tree in the wind, steady and sure no matter what the outside circumstances may be. Tree Pose stretches the thighs, groins, torso, and shoulders. It builds strength in the ankles and calves, and it tones the abdominal muscles.

In order to fully gain the meditative benefits of Tree Pose, it's important to stay grounded and calm in the pose, while still maintaining alignment. Here are a couple of tips to help you stand up as tall as a tree:

- Take your time. As with any balancing pose, it's often easier to come into the pose slowly and with awareness. If you enter the pose quickly, you are more likely to lose your balance, which makes it more difficult to regain your balance once it's lost.

- Don't worry if you fall over. Just set up and start again.

- Mountain Pose provides the structural foundation for Tree Pose. Be sure you know how to do Mountain Pose before attempting Tree Pose.

- Work the pose from the ground up. Balance your weight entirely across your standing foot— across the inner and outer ankles, big toe and baby toe. Then, bring your awareness to the shin, calf, and thigh of your standing leg. Find alignment in your hips, tailbone, pelvis, and belly, and then in your collarbones, shoulder blades, arms, and neck. Extend the pose through the crown of your head. When you are ready, you can *then* raise your arms overhead.

- Never rest the foot of your raised leg directly on your knee or at the side of your knee joint!

- To help with balancing, bring your awareness to the center line of your body—the vertical line that runs directly through the center of your head, neck, and torso.

- Like a tree, extend your roots down and blossom your arms up toward the sun. The stronger the roots, the taller the tree.

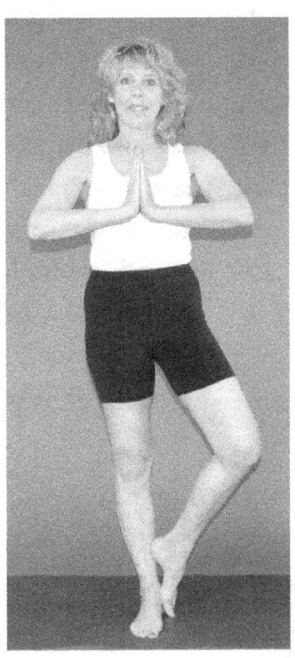

Variation: If you have difficulty balancing on one foot to start, place the toes of the other foot on the ground until you gain better balance.

Tree Pose improves your sense of balance and coordination. Regular practice will improve your focus and your ability to concentrate in all areas of your life, particularly during those times when you might normally feel "off balance." This pose has a positive impact on the grace and

139

ease with which you approach all circumstances, even outside your yoga class. It teaches the benefits of a meditative state of mind and is a gentle reminder that you can bring calm focus and clear-headedness to all situations, *not* just when you are practicing a seated meditation.

How to do it:

1. Begin standing in Mountain Pose, with your arms at your sides. Distribute your weight evenly across both feet, grounding down equally through your inner ankles, outer ankles, big toes, and baby toes.

2. Shift your weight to your left foot. Bend your right knee, then reach down and clasp your right inner ankle. Use your hand to draw your right foot alongside your inner left thigh. If you cannot put your foot that high, rest the arch against the calf. If even that is too difficult, place your arch over the ankle bone. The height of the foot is not important; do not let the pose be about how high you can get your bent leg. Also, never rest your foot against your knee, only above or below it. Adjust your position so the center of your pelvis is directly over your left foot.

3. Rest your hands on your hips and lengthen your tailbone toward the floor. Then press your palms together in prayer position at your chest, with your thumbs resting on your sternum.

4. Fix your gaze gently on one unmoving point in front of you. Create steadiness here.

5. Press your standing leg into the ground. Press your right foot into your left thigh (or wherever it is) while pressing your thigh (or calf) firmly against that foot.

6. Inhale as you slowly extend your arms overhead, reaching your fingertips to the sky as a tree reaches its branches. Rotate your palms inward to face each other. If your shoulders are more flexible, you can press your palms together in prayer position overhead. You can separate your arms slightly. Energize your arms by engaging your triceps muscles.

7. Hold for up to one minute. To release the pose, step back into Mountain Pose. Repeat for the same amount of time on the opposite side.

Modifications & Variations

Practicing Tree Pose can be a great way to gain balance, grace, and poise—for beginners *and* advanced students. Try these simple changes to adapt the pose to your current abilities:

- If you are unable to bring your foot to your thigh, rest your foot alongside your calf muscle or the ankle of your standing leg instead. Rest the toes of your raised foot on the floor if you need assistance balancing.

- If you are very unsteady, try practicing the pose with your back against a wall for extra support. Alternatively, you can place a chair next to the standing-leg side of your body and rest your hand on the back of the chair for extra support. Practicing this balance pose, even with assistance, gives great benefit.

For a greater challenge, when your arms are overhead, practice balancing without using the outside world for reference by closing your eyes.

HALF-MOON POSE (ARDHA CHANDRASANA)

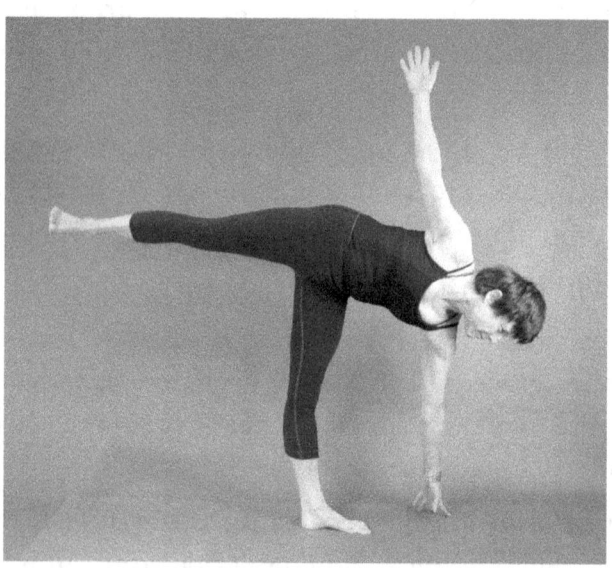

Half Moon Pose is a standing yoga posture that will challenge your leg muscles and your ability to balance. It is a fun and exhilarating pose, which can be easily transitioned into from Triangle Pose. The two poses are similar in their full-body extension; Half Moon is like a balancing variation of Triangle.

There are a variety of modifications available for this pose, making it a suitable balancing posture for beginning and advanced yoga students.

Half Moon Pose strengthens the thighs, ankles, abdomen, and buttocks. It opens the chest, shoulders, and torso, while lengthening the spine. This pose also effectively stretches the groins, hamstrings, and calves.

Because your head is lower than your heart in Half Moon, this pose also provides the benefits of a mild inversion, including reduction of stress, anxiety, and fatigue. Half Moon also stimulates the organs of the torso, which can provide relief from digestive distress, such as indigestion and constipation.

Most notably, Half Moon improves your sense of balance and full-body coordination. It helps to increase your body awareness and the sense of your body's position in space (this sense is called proprioception). Improving your proprioception can bring more poise to your everyday activities. It can also help you prevent the risk of falls and injuries by making you more aware of your body's position and movements.

Caution: Do not practice Half Moon Pose if you have low blood pressure or are currently experiencing headaches, insomnia, or diarrhea. Those with neck injuries should not turn their heads to face the top hand, but should continue looking straight ahead.

How to do it:

1. Begin by standing at the top of your mat. Turn to the left and step your feet wide apart. Extend your arms out to the sides at shoulder-height. Your feet should be as far apart as your wrists. Rotate your right (front) foot ninety degrees so your front foot's toes point to the top of the mat. Turn your left foot's toes slightly in. Align your front heel with the arch of your back foot.

2. Reach through your right hand in the same direction that your right foot is pointed. Shift your left hip back and then fold sideways at the hip. Rest your right hand on your outer right shin or ankle. If you are more flexible, place your fingertips on the floor. You can also place your hand on a yoga block.

3. Align your shoulders so your left shoulder is directly above your right shoulder. If flexible enough, turn your head to gaze at your left thumb; if not, look down at your right hand. This is Extended Triangle Pose.

4. Bring your left hand to rest on your left hip. Turn your head to look at the floor. Then, bend your right knee and step your left foot six to twelve inches closer to your right foot. Place your right

hand's fingertips on the floor in front of your right foot and about six inches to the right of your foot.

5. Press firmly into your right hand and foot. Straighten your right leg while simultaneously lifting your left leg. Work toward bringing your left leg parallel to the floor or even higher than your hips.

6. Reach actively through your left heel. Do not lock your right leg's knee. Keep your right foot's toes and kneecap facing toward the front of the mat.

7. Stack your top hip directly over your bottom hip, and open your torso to the left. Then extend your left arm and point your fingertips toward the sky. If you can balance comfortably there, turn your head and gaze at your left thumb. (This is challenging to your balance—beginners, continue looking at your right foot.)

8. Draw your shoulder blades firmly into your back. Lengthen your tailbone toward your left heel.

9. Breathe and hold for up to one minute. To release, lower your left leg as you exhale. Return to Extended Triangle Pose. Inhale and press firmly through your left heel as you lift your torso. Lower your arms. Turn to the left, reversing the position of your feet, and repeat for the same length of time on the opposite side.

Practicing Half Moon Pose will strengthen and

stretch your entire body. It can sometimes be difficult for beginners to find balance and correct alignment. Try these simple modifications to find a variation of the pose that works for you:

- If you can't touch the floor with your bottom hand or fingertips, rest your hand on a block. Begin with the block on its highest side. Gradually lower it to the middle, and then to its lowest height as you gain more confidence.

- Beginners can practice this pose with their backs against a wall. This will provide support and ease any fear of falling as you learn the correct alignment of the pose.

CROW POSE (BAKASANA)

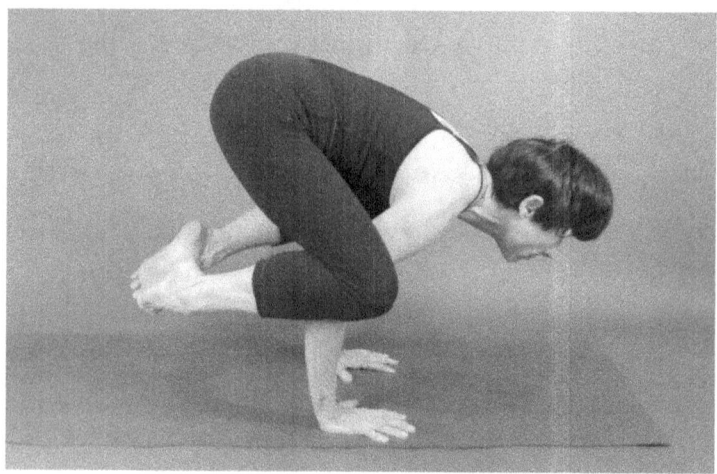

Crow Pose (also sometimes called Crane Pose) is usually the first arm balance that yoga students learn.

It is the foundational pose for most arm balances in yoga, so it's a good idea to understand the basics of Crow Pose first. Though it may seem tricky, Crow can be a fun pose when you get the hang of it. Practicing Crow Pose can be a great way to challenge your mind! It requires less physical strength than you might imagine. The real challenge is in your mindset.

Crow Pose strengthens the upper arms, forearms, and wrists. Additionally, it tones and strengthens the abdominal muscles and the organs of the torso while stretching the upper back and groins. This pose also improves balance and full-body coordination.

More significantly, Crow Pose builds confidence and healthy self-awareness. Getting over the fear of possibly falling on your face requires moving slowly with a calm mind. This focused mindset will help you reduce everyday stress and anxiety, leaving you feeling calm and self-assured.

This pose requires a good deal of strength, so it is often performed closer to the beginning of a yoga session. Be sure to warm up thoroughly with several Sun Salutations before attempting Crow.

Caution: Do not practice this pose if you have a recent or chronic wrist or shoulder injury, or if you have carpal tunnel syndrome. Women who are pregnant should also avoid this pose.

This pose requires a bit of confidence, but it is not

difficult so much as tricky. Don't get discouraged if you can't do it on the first try, and remember that everyone learning this pose falls! (But being so low to the ground, you don't have far to go.) Newer students might feel more comfortable doing the pose with a pile of blankets or a pillow in front of them in case they fall forward. Be sure to set up your "falling spot" before you start practicing the pose.

How to do it:

Begin by standing at the top of your mat in Mountain Pose, with your arms at your sides. Step your feet about as wide as your mat.

Bend your knees and lower your hips, coming into a squat. Separate your thighs so they are slightly wider than your torso, keep your heels as close to the floor as possible. If your heels lift, that's okay.

Crow Preparation: Start in Squatting Prayer Pose, then lean forward and place hands on floor.

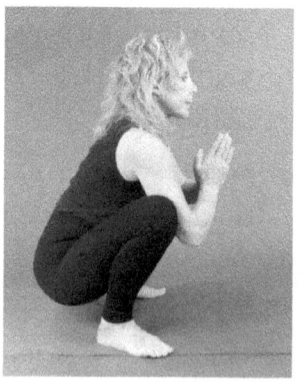
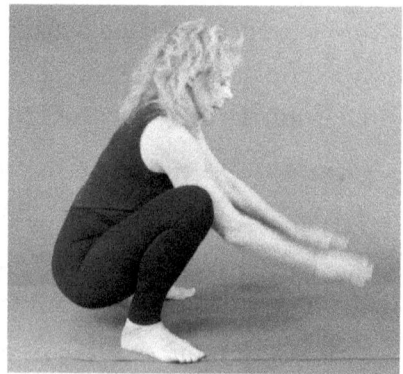

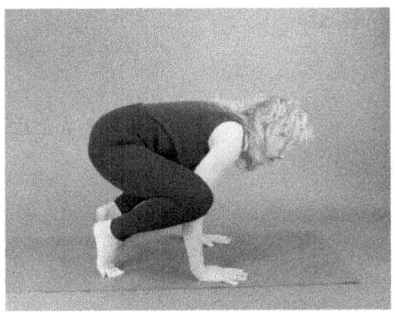

Drop your torso slightly forward and bring your upper arms to the inside of your knees. Press your elbows along the inside of your knees and bring your palms to the mat, keeping them about shoulder-distance apart. Spread your fingers and press evenly across both palms and through your knuckles.

Press your shins against the back of your upper arms. Draw your knees in as close to your underarms as possible.

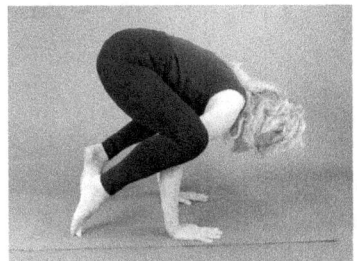 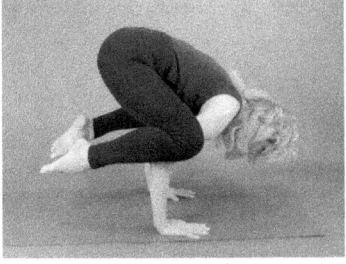

Lift onto the balls of your feet as you lean forward. Round your back and draw your abdominal muscles in firmly. Keep your tailbone tucked in toward your heels.

Look at the floor about twelve inches in front of your hands, or at a point even more forward if possible.

As you continue to lean on your hands and shift your weight forward, lift your feet off the floor and draw your heels toward your buttocks. If it's difficult to lift both feet at the same time, try lifting one foot and then the other. Balance your torso and legs on the back of your upper arms.

Keep pressing evenly across your palms and fingers, then begin to straighten your elbows. Keep your knees and shins hugging in tightly toward your armpits. Keep your forearms drawn firmly toward the midline of your body.

Hold the pose for up to one minute. To release, exhale as you slowly lower your feet to the floor, coming back into a squat. Then rotate your knees down, sit back on your heels, and rest in Child's Pose for a minute.

Crow Pose can be fun and uplifting, but it's important not to let yourself get frustrated if you fall out of it. Keep in mind that *everyone* falls when learning this pose!

WARRIOR POSE III (VIRABHADRASANA III)

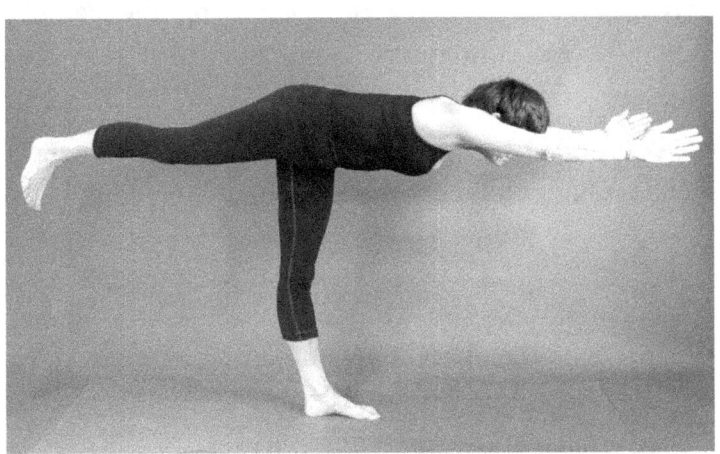

Warrior Pose III is an intermediate balancing pose. This dynamic standing posture creates stability throughout your entire body by integrating all of the muscles throughout your core, arms, and legs. Practicing Warrior III will build balance and strength. It might take some time to be able to balance for more than a breath or two, so remember to move at your own pace. Don't be afraid to fall out of the pose. Take it slowly—stability will come with practice.

Warrior III strengthens the whole back side of the body, including the shoulders, thighs, calves, ankles, and back. It also tones and strengthens the abdominal muscles. Warrior III improves balance, posture, and full-body coordination.

This pose also enhances your ability to concentrate, keeping your mind calmly focused when faced with difficulty. Learning to hone your attention while staying serene is a key to discovering the connection between your mind, body, and spirit—the true meaning of yoga.

Caution: Do not practice this pose if you are experiencing high blood pressure or heart problems.

How to do it:

1. Begin standing in Mountain Pose with your feet hip-distance apart and your arms at your sides. Breathe smoothly and calmly, bringing your awareness to the present moment.

2. Turn to the left and step your feet wide apart, about four to five feet. Turn your right foot out ninety degrees so your toes point toward the top of the mat. Pivot your left foot inward at a forty-five-degree angle. Point your pelvis and torso in the same direction as your right toes are pointing.

3. Bend your right knee over your right ankle so your shin is perpendicular to the floor. Raise your arms overhead with your palms facing each other. This is Warrior Pose I.

4. Press your weight into your right foot. Lift your left leg as you lower your torso, bringing your body parallel to the ground. Your arms, still extended, will now reach forward.

5. Flex your left foot and reach out through your heel, as if you're pressing a wall behind you.

6. Keep the muscles of both legs actively engaged. Straighten your standing leg as you continue to lift the left leg, but do not lock your knees.

7. Work toward bringing your arms, torso, hips, and raised leg parallel to the floor. You may need to lower the hip of your raised leg slightly in order to bring your hips parallel to your mat.

8. Stretch your body from your fingertips all the way through your lifted heel.

9. Gaze at the floor a few feet in front of your body.

10. Hold the pose for thirty seconds. To release, exhale as you softly lower your left foot back to the floor, coming again into Warrior I. Lower your arms and step forward into Mountain Pose. Repeat the pose for the same amount of time on the opposite side.

Modifications & Variations

Try this simple change to find a variation of the pose that works best for you:

If you are having difficulty balancing, try practicing the pose with a wall or chair at an arm's distance in front of you. Then lightly rest your hands on the wall or chair for support.

Keep these tips in mind:

- Do not lock or hyperextend the knee of your standing leg. Resist your standing-leg calf muscle against the shin; this micro-movement will stabilize your lower leg.

- Do not bring your raised leg higher than your hips or your head. Work to keep your arms, trunk, and raised leg in one line and parallel to the ground.

- Keep your spine in one straight line with your neck relaxed, not stiff or compressed. Reach forward through the crown of your head.

- Strongly engage your leg muscles.

- Draw your abdominal muscles in toward your spine. This will help to protect your lower back.

- Focus on the stretch, not on the lift! It doesn't matter how high your leg goes if you don't have correct alignment. Work toward maintaining an equal balance of energy and effort in both legs.

STANDING THIGH STRETCH
(PREPARATION FOR LORD OF THE DANCE POSE)

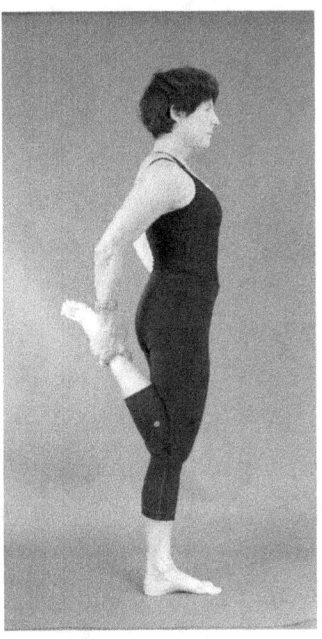

The quadriceps—the group of four muscles on the front of your thigh—make up some of the strongest muscles in your body. Quads are the primary mover in any bent-leg activity, including cycling, hiking, climbing stairs, and running. But they also get worked in many yoga poses, like Warrior I and II.

Standing Thigh Stretch lengthens and adds flexibility to these powerhouse muscles. It's a great pose to practice after standing yoga postures. It also helps prepare the body for poses that require mobile hip flexors (front hip joints) and quadriceps.

Be sure to warm up your legs before practicing this pose. Stretching your quads when the muscles are cold can lead to strained knees and deep muscle tears. Some good warm-ups include the sequence of Sun Salutation followed by Crescent Lunge.

Standing Thigh Stretch improves flexibility in the quadriceps and hip flexors. It also helps release tension in the lower back and hips. This pose soothes stiffness in the spine and legs, and improves posture. It also tones the abdominal muscles.

While it's important to keep your quadriceps strong, it's equally important to keep them flexible! Regularly stretching your quads will prevent them from becoming short and tight, a condition that limits your range of motion. Keeping your thighs and hip flexors mobile reduces your chance of injury while also preventing post-workout soreness. Since the human body works holistically (as an integrated system), flexible quads and hip flexors also help prevent knee, hip, and lower-back pain.

Caution: If you have a knee injury or arthritis, only attempt this pose under the guidance of an experienced and knowledgeable instructor.

How to do it:

1. Stand in Mountain Pose with your feet together and your arms at your sides.
2. Shift your weight onto your left foot.

3. Bend your right knee and bring your right heel toward your right buttock. Reach your right hand down and clasp your right ankle. Relax your left hand at your side or place it on your left hip if you need help with balancing. (If you need more help to balance, rest your left hand on a heavy chair.)

4. Push your right hip slightly forward and your knee slightly back. Try to align your right knee directly under your right hip, while keeping your right and left hips in line with each other. Keep your knees close together; do not let your right knee slide open to the side.

5. Stand up straight. Draw your abdominal muscles in and up, point your tailbone toward the floor, and be sure not to arch your back. Keep your shoulders relaxed.

6. Hold here, breathing for up to thirty seconds.

7. To release, gently let go of your ankle and step your right foot to the floor. Stand in Mountain Pose for a moment. Repeat the pose on the opposite side for the same length of time.

Keep these things in mind:

- Standing Thigh Stretch can open up the front side of your lower body when done in correct alignment. It's important to come into the pose slowly. Use props (chair, strap) as needed, and make whatever modifications you need to feel safe and supported as you gain flexibility. Regularly practicing Standing Thigh Stretch will gradually result in greater flexibility and strength. As you become more comfortable in the pose, you may also notice improved posture and stronger core muscles!

- If you can't hold onto your ankle or foot, use a strap. Wrap a yoga strap around the top of your foot, then bend your knee and come into the pose. Hold onto both ends of the strap with your same-side hand.

- Be very careful not to strain your bent knee. If you experience any knee pain, lower your foot immediately and come out of the pose. Knee injuries take a long time to heal, and you can permanently damage your ligaments if you force yourself into this pose before you are ready. Don't pull, push, or force any movement in this pose. Let your movements be slow and smooth.

- Keep the knee and toes of your standing leg facing directly forward.

- Keep the muscles of your standing leg engaged, and do not lock your knee.

LORD OF THE DANCE POSE (NATARAJASANA)

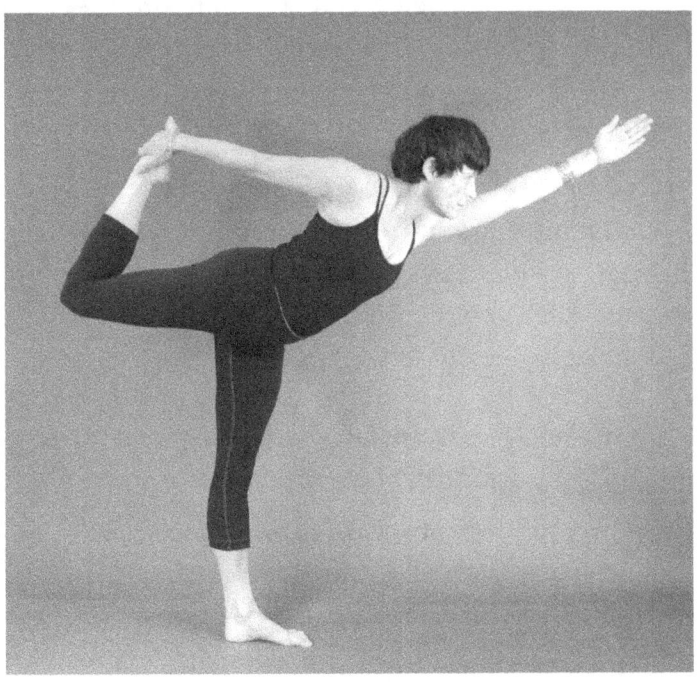

Lord of the Dance Pose is an intermediate, standing yoga pose that combines the challenging aspects of balancing with a backbend. This pose requires and builds full-body strength, flexibility, and coordination. It opens the shoulders, chest, and hips as it stretches and strengthens the thighs, ankles, and abdomen, while it also develops greater flexibility in your spine, shoulders, and hamstrings. It also stretches the entire front of the body while strengthening the back muscles, which improves posture.

Not the least notably, Lord of the Dance pose

gives you the ability to concentrate and focus while at the same time balancing and stretching into a rather significant backbend. The ability to remain calm and centered in this pose will improve your poise, grace, and focus in daily life.

Caution: Do not practice this pose if you have a recent or chronic ankle or low back injury. Also avoid this pose if you are currently experiencing low blood pressure, dizziness, or migraines.

How to do it:

1. Stand in Mountain Pose with your feet together and your arms at your sides.

2. Shift your weight onto your left foot. Make sure that your weight is spread out across all four corners of your foot.

3. Firm up the muscles in your left leg, but do not lock out the knee.

4. Bend your right knee and bring your right heel up toward your right buttock. Reach your right hand down and clasp that ankle. You can also loop a strap or towel around the top of your right foot and then hold onto the strap with your right hand. Pull your knees together.

5. Reach your left arm overhead, pointing your fingertips toward the ceiling. If your balance is shaky, place your hand on a chair in front of you.

6. Fix your gaze softly at an unmoving spot in front of you. Make sure your left kneecap and toes continue to point directly forward.

7. When you feel steady and comfortable, and only then, begin to press your right foot away from your body as you simultaneously pivot on your left hip and lean your torso slightly forward. Keep your chest lifting and continue reaching your left fingertips up toward the ceiling. Go slowly and maintain control of the pose. It is not important how far you raise your leg.

8. Raise your right foot as high as you can. At the same time, pull in your abs and press your tailbone toward the floor to avoid compressing your lower back. Do not let your right knee fly open to the side.

9. As you press your raised foot back, keep your chest lifting. Do not let your torso drop too far forward. Keep your pelvis facing front and your right knee drawn in toward the midline of your body.

10. If you are holding a strap, gradually make the strap shorter until your hand is close to your foot.

11. Hold for five breaths. To release, very slowly and gently return to your starting position. Then lower your right foot and come back into Mountain Pose. Repeat the pose on the opposite side for the same amount of time.

Modifications & Variations

Lord of the Dance Pose can be a great way to gain flexibility, strength, and poise. Be sure to modify the pose as needed and ease up if you feel any pinching or jarring pain, especially in your back or neck. Here are a few simple modifications that will lighten or deepen the pose for you:

- If you can't hold onto the ankle of your raised leg, use a strap. Wrap a yoga strap around the top of your foot, then bend your knee and come into the pose. Hold onto both ends of the strap with your same-side hand.

- If you are brand new to the pose, practice Standing Thigh Stretch to gain the flexibility and strength needed for this pose.

- If it's difficult to balance, rest your free hand on a wall, chair, or any other stable object.

Practicing Lord of the Dance pose will benefit you in body, mind, and spirit. Keep the following information in mind when practicing this pose:

- Keep your gaze fixed on an unmoving spot in front of you.

- Make sure your bent knee does not splay open to the side.

- Keep the knee and toes of your standing leg facing directly forward.

- Firm the muscles of your standing leg, but do not lock or hyperextend your knee. Resist your standing-leg calf muscle against the shin; this micro-movement will stabilize your lower leg.

- Keep your neck relaxed, not stiff or compressed. Reach forward through the crown of your head.

- Evenly distribute the backbend across your upper, middle, and lower back.

- Keep breathing throughout the pose. Do not hold your breath.

- Move slowly and don't be afraid to fall! If you do fall, simply set up and start again.

BIG TOE POSE (PADANGUSTHASANA)

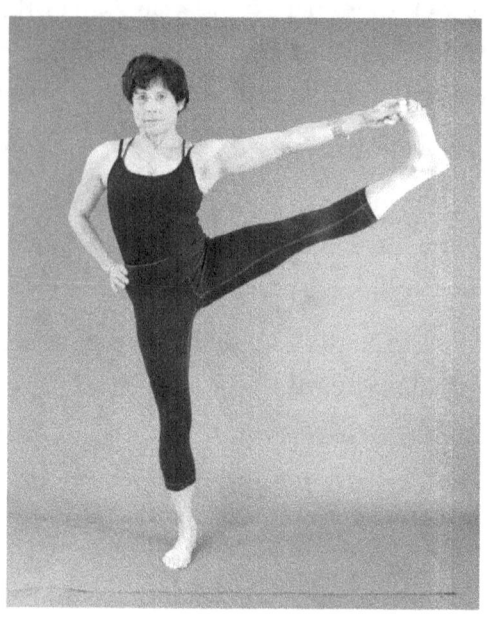

Another intermediate standing balance pose, Big Toe Pose is not difficult to do once you get your center of gravity correct. It's a fun pose to do and very satisfying once you are able to balance in it. This pose requires flexibility in the hip joints and back strength, and it will increase your ability to concentrate. It's more important to keep your spine straight and your shoulders relaxed than it is to straighten your lifted leg. You can keep your lifted leg bent, or use a strap if you need to, but be sure your spine stays tall and upright throughout the pose.

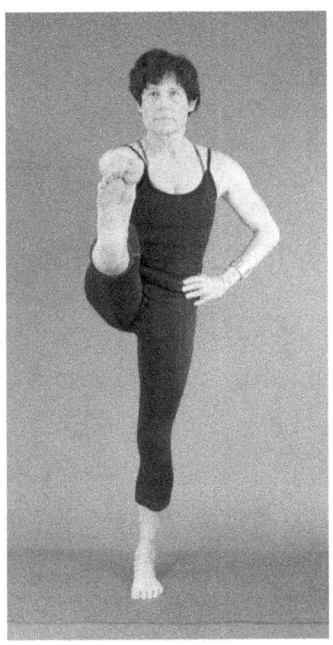

How to do it:

1. Begin in Mountain Pose with your feet together and arms at your sides. Place your left hand on your left hip. Breathe deeply and draw your awareness to the present moment.

2. Shift your weight to your left foot. Slowly draw your right knee up toward your chest. Bring your right arm to the inside of your right thigh. Then loop the first two fingers around your right foot's big toe, holding onto them with your thumb. Stretch the crown of your head up toward the ceiling.

3. Straighten your spine. Strongly engage your abdominal muscles and the muscles of your left leg. Straighten your left leg, but do not lock your knee.

4. On an exhalation, begin to extend your right leg forward. Straighten your right leg as much as possible. Use a strap around your foot if needed, and make any other adjustments to ensure that you're not pushing yourself too hard in this pose. Be patient. You will gain flexibility in time.

5. Keep both hips squared forward and keep your spine straight. Keep your shoulders and neck soft and relaxed.

6. Drop your right hip slightly so it is in line with your left hip. Bring your awareness to your midline— the line that runs directly down the center of your body.

7. Hold for five to ten breaths. To release, draw your knee back into your chest, then slowly lower your foot to the floor. Come back to Mountain Pose. Then repeat on the opposite side for the same amount of time.

BOAT POSE (NAVASANA)

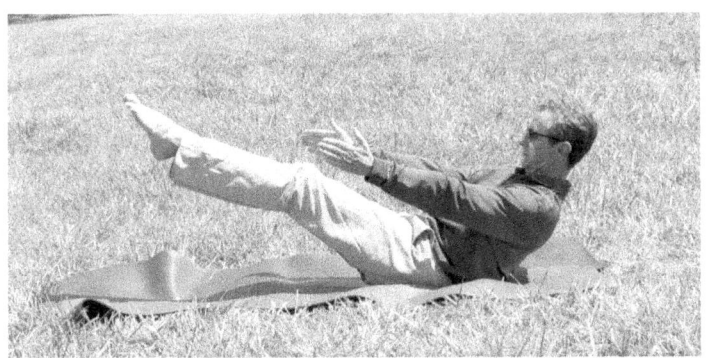

One of the best core-strengthening poses, Boat Pose requires strength and balance. This pose works the total front side of the body, including the abdomen, back, chest, shoulders, arms, and thighs.

Boat Pose deeply challenges the abdomen, spine, and hip flexors, building strength and steadiness at the body's core. It stimulates the abdominal organs, including the kidneys and intestines, which improves digestion. This pose also encourages healthy regulation of the thyroid and prostate glands, helping to maintain metabolism and relieve stress. It's more important to keep your spine straight and the front of your torso long than it is to straighten your legs or balance without hand support. Keep your hands on the floor and knees bent until you have built up enough strength to deepen the pose while keeping proper alignment.

Often strenuous at first, this pose requires (and

helps further develop) concentration and stamina. Practicing Boat Pose regularly will increase your ability to stay focused, internally aware, and emotionally calm.

One of the tricky things in this pose is that you need to breathe while you are contracting your stomach muscles, which forces you to engage the intercostal muscles in between the ribs to expand the rib cage while breathing.

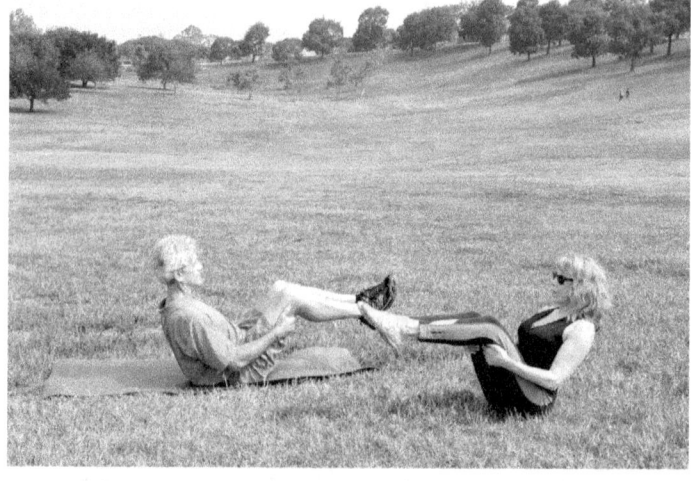

Modifications: Those with heart problems and asthma should not practice the full variation of the pose, but should gradually and gently practice assisted Boat Pose (see photo above) instead. Women who are pregnant should not practice Boat Pose. Those with back injuries can practice this pose with their backs or heads supported against a wall to gain strength.

As you gain strength, you can lift your hands and clasp your outer thighs. Eventually, you will be able to extend your arms forward and straighten your legs.

How to do it:

1. Begin seated with your knees bent and feet flat on the floor, hands resting beside your hips. Draw your awareness inward and focus on your breath. Allow your inhalations and exhalations to be smooth, calm, and even.

2. Keeping your spine straight, lean back slightly and lift your feet, bringing your shins parallel to the floor.

3. Draw in your low back, lift your chest, and lengthen the front of your torso. Then extend your arms forward, in line with your shoulders with your palms facing each other.

4. Balance on your sit bones, keeping your spine straight. Take care not to let your lower back sag or your chest collapse.

5. Lengthen the front of your torso from your pubic bone to the top of your sternum. The lower belly (the area below your navel) should be firm and somewhat flat, but not hard or thick.

6. With an exhale, straighten your legs to a forty-five-degree angle from the ground, bringing your body into a V shape.

7. Keep your breath easy, steady, and smooth. Focus your awareness within. Soften your eyes and your face. Gaze at your toes.

8. Spread your shoulder blades wide and reach out through your fingers, actively engaging your hands.

9. Stay in the pose for five breaths, gradually working up to one minute. To release the pose, exhale as you lower your legs and hands to the floor.

Things to remember:

As you gain strength, you can lift your hands and clasp your outer thighs. Eventually, you will be able to extend your arms forward and straighten your legs.

If your hamstrings are tight, it can be difficult to straighten your legs. Keep your knees bent and work on building core strength first.

For assistance straightening your legs, wrap a strap around the soles of both feet. Hold the strap firmly with both hands. As you inhale, lean your torso back. Exhaling, press your feet against the strap as you lift and lengthen your legs.

If you'd like more of a challenge in Full Boat Pose, lightly clasp your hands behind your head. With an exhalation, slightly lower your legs while also lowering your back a few inches toward the floor. Inhale to lift up again into the full pose.

SIDE PLANK POSE (VASISTHASANA)

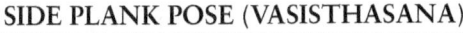

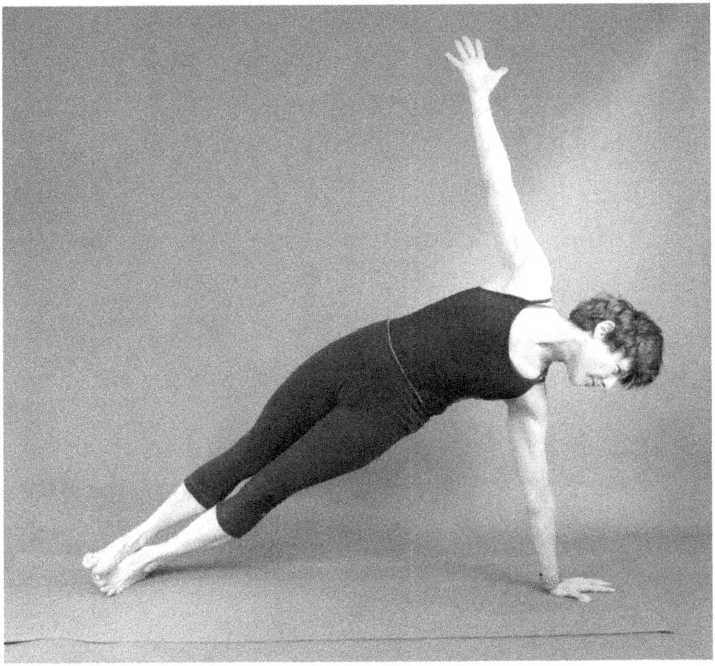

A powerful arm balance, Side Plank Pose challenges your ability to stay calm and focused. This pose strengthens your wrists, forearms, shoulders, and spine. It increases flexibility in the wrists and the full variation also opens the hips and hamstrings. This pose tones the abdominal muscles and improves balance, concentration, and focus.

Side Plank Pose requires a lot of strength to be performed correctly. It is very easy to injure yourself if you move into it too soon. If you do not yet have the strength to do the pose in proper alignment, practice the pose with your lower knee on the floor. (See photo above for modified version.) Side Plank Pose can build arm and core strength quickly. However, it's vital to ensure you are performing the pose with correct alignment; otherwise you can easily injure your shoulders, elbows, and wrists.

Caution: Avoid this pose if you have an arm, shoulder, or wrist injury.

How to do it:

1. Begin in Downward Facing Dog. Lower your hips and shift your weight forward to come into Plank Pose (the top of a push-up): palms flat, body extended, with your legs reaching through your heels.

2. Step your feet together and press your weight down through your right hand and forearm. Then, roll your body to the right, balancing on the outer edge of your right foot. Stack your left foot on top of your right foot and keep your legs straight.

3. Beginners can modify by lowering their right knee and shin to the mat, keeping their hips lifted while building strength in the arms and torso.

4. Extend your left arm to the sky, reaching through your fingertips as you lift your hips and firm the triceps of both arms. Feel the muscles across your shoulder blades flex. Firm your thighs, and press through your heels into the floor.

5. Bring your body into one straight line. Gaze at your top thumb. Press down through your bottom index finger.

6. Hold for up to thirty seconds. Exhale as you slowly return to Plank Pose, then into Downward Facing Dog. Repeat on the opposite side. After both sides, rest in Child's Pose.

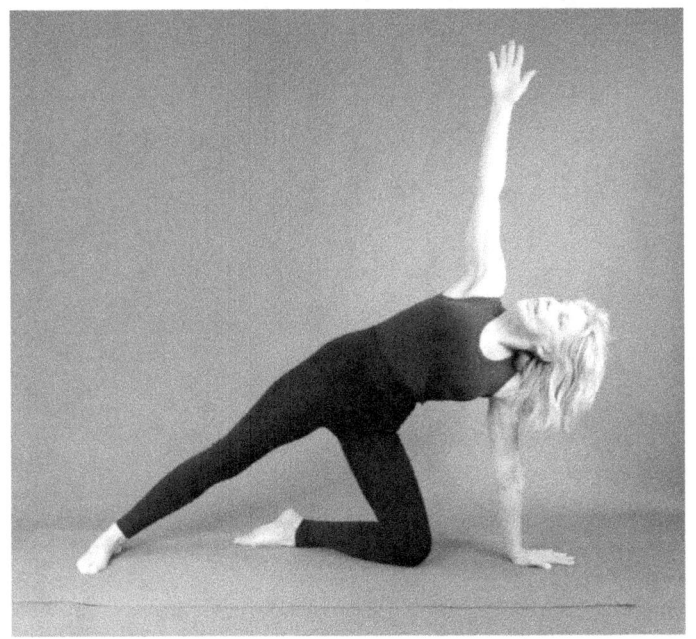

Modification: Place the knee of the lower leg on the mat.

Side Plank Pose is a powerful arm and core strengthener when practiced correctly. However, it takes time to gain enough strength to hold the pose for more than a breath or two. Remember to take it slowly and be careful not to strain your arms, wrists, elbows, or shoulders.

Try these simple changes for a variation that might be more suitable for you:

- Don't forget you can always bring your bottom knee and shin to the mat until you have enough strength to fully support your body weight on your arm.

- For a variation of the previous modification, keep your bottom leg extended, bend your top knee, and step your top foot in front of your body.

CHAPTER 7

Yoga Sequences

In the pages that follow, you will find suggested sequences for practicing your yoga sessions, grouped according to the attribute that the pose will develop—flexibility, stamina, balance, or fat burning. Of course, all of the poses overlap categories to a large extent. For example, Standing Splits Pose not only works on developing balance but also requires strength and flexibility as well. So even if you are doing the balance sequence, rest assured you are working on all the other qualities you wish to develop, including stamina, strength, and relaxation.

Not every pose needs to be done in every session, but since these are such important and effective poses, every pose should be done at least once a week (twice a week is preferable).

If you practice every day, mix up the sequences so that you are not doing the same poses every time. There are warm-up poses that should be done at every session, including Child's Pose, Cat-Cow Pose, and Sun Salutations, as well as cool-down poses, including Corpse Pose, but feel free to mix up the postures in any way you feel is right.

Remember to not overdo it as you are starting out. Listen to your body and rest between poses in Child's Pose if you like.

SUN SALUTATION WARM-UP FOR YOGA SEQUENCES

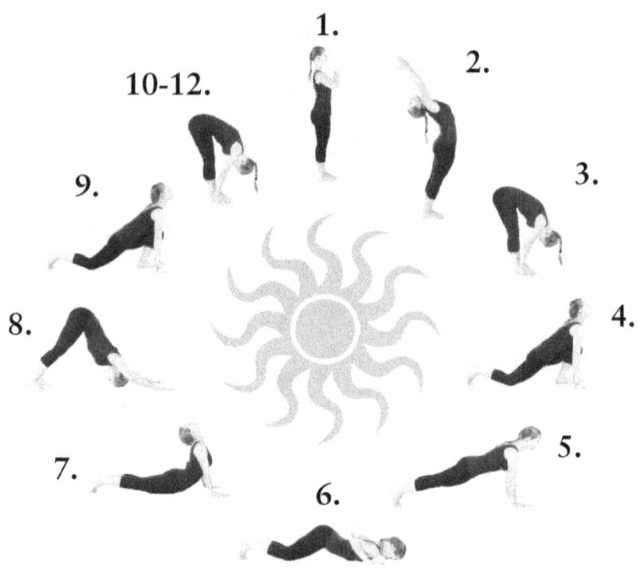

The Sun Salutation (Surya Namaskar) is done to warm up the body because Sun Salutations touches upon all the major muscles that you'll be using in your practice. You have already been introduced to each one of the parts. Done in a sequence, it is like a flowing dance coordinating each movement with the breath. You can watch a simple video of this sequence at YogaJournal.com.

How to do it:

1. Start out standing with your palms together in front of your heart. Do deep ocean sound breathing (Ujjayi) here for a moment (breathe in and out through your nose, close up your throat

slightly so that the breath makes a sound in your throat). Then begin:

2. Inhaling, straighten out your elbows, drop your hands down, and with your hands clasped, raise hands overhead, sweeping your arms up as high as you can, upper arms next to your ears. If it feels good to you, bend back slightly here to stretch out the front of the body. Press your hips forward, lift your chest to open, and tighten your buttocks.

3. Exhaling, dive forward in a graceful swan dive to forward fold, fingertips either on the floor even with your toes or place your hands on your shins. Then place the hands on the floor on either side of your feet, bending the knees as much as needed if you are not flexible enough to put your palms on the floor with your legs straight.

4. Inhaling, move your right foot back to high lunge position, toes pointing toward your hands. On the ball of the foot, pressing back heel backward, lengthen your spine.

5. Retaining the breath, bring your left foot back to meet the right, coming into plank pose. Hands flat on the floor, directly under your shoulders, legs straight, resting on the balls of the feet, toes pointing toward your hands. Try to get your body in one straight line from your shoulders to your heels, not sagging down too much or humping up.

6. Exhaling, lower your entire body to the mat, with your hands next to your rib cage, palms flat. Put the tops of your feet on the floor.

7. Inhaling, keeping the elbows close to the body and your hips on the floor, press your shoulders back and down, and gently lift your upper body off the mat. Tops of the feet are on the floor. Look forward or upward if that feels comfortable.

8. Tuck your toes under and, exhaling, lift your tailbone up toward the ceiling into Downward Facing Dog. Feet and hands about shoulder width apart, try to straighten your legs and arms. Point your tailbone up and use your arm and shoulder strength to press your body back toward your legs.

9. Inhaling, bring your right leg forward and come into high lunge with the left leg back, up on the ball of the left foot.

10. Exhaling, bring the left foot forward, and come into forward bend.

11. Inhaling, sweep your hands and arms up overhead, standing up, and come into a slight backward bend, opening your chest, and push your pelvis forward. Lengthen your spine.

12. Exhaling, bring your hands together in front of your heart and stand upright in Mountain Pose.

RELAXATION AND FLEXIBILITY SEQUENCE

POSE	Name Amount of time you should stay in pose
	Child's Pose One to two minutes, center yourself and breathe.
	Cat–Cow Stretch Ten times – Arch and flex, with breathing.
	Sun Salutations Three or four rounds to get warmed up. Be sure to "marry" each movement with either an inhale or an exhale.
	Forward Bend – One minute. Remember to use props if needed.
	Side Bends – Three to five breaths per side.
	Back Bending – Three to five breaths.

	Bound Angle Pose and/or Reclining Bound Angle Pose – One to five minutes; if reclining, as long as you like.
	Pigeon Pose with body upright or lying down over front leg – One to two minutes per side.
	Spinal Twists with straight or bent leg – Three to five breaths per side.
	Happy Baby Pose – One minute.
	Plow Pose – Three to five breaths, or if you prefer not to do this pose, go to Legs up the Wall Pose.
	Legs up the Wall Pose – As long as you like.
	Corpse Pose – Five to twenty minutes.

STAMINA SEQUENCE

POSE	Name Amount of time you should stay in pose
	Child's Pose One to two minutes, center yourself and breathe.
	Cat–Cow Stretch Ten times – Arch and flex, with breathing.
	Sun Salutations Three or four rounds to get warmed up. Be sure to "marry" each movement with either an inhale or an exhale.
	Downward Facing Dog Pose One minute.
	Upward Facing Dog Pose – One minute.
	Mountain Pose – Three to five breaths.
	Warrior I Pose – Three to five breaths, each side.

	Warrior II Pose – Three to five breaths, each side.
	Triangle Pose – Three to five breaths, each side.
	Revolved Triangle Pose – Three to five breaths, each side.
	Chair Pose – Five breaths.
	Plank Pose – Five to ten breaths.
	Boat Pose – Three to five breaths.
	Shoulder Stand – One to five minutes.

	Happy Baby Pose – One minute.
	Child's Pose – One minute.
	Corpse Pose – Five to twenty minutes.

BALANCE SEQUENCE

POSE	Name and amount of time you should stay in pose
	Child's Pose One to two minutes, center yourself and breathe.
	Cat–Cow Stretch Ten times – Arch and flex, with breathing.
	Sun Salutations Three or four rounds to get warmed up. Be sure to "marry" each movement with either an inhale or an exhale.
	Downward Facing Dog Pose – One minute.
	Upward Facing Dog Pose – One minute.
	Mountain Pose – Three to five breaths.
	Hand to Toe Pose – Three to five breaths, each side.

	Thigh Stretch Three to five breaths, each side.
	Lord of the Dance Pose Three to five breaths, each side.
	Standing Splits One minute or five breaths.
	Warrior III – Five breaths.
	Eagle Pose Three to five breaths, each side.
	Tree Pose Thirty seconds to one minute balancing.
	Side Plank Pose Five to ten breaths, each side.

	Crow Pose – Thirty seconds.
	Boat Pose – Three to five breaths.
	Shoulder Stand – One to five minutes.
	Happy Baby Pose – One minute.
	Child's Pose – One minute.
	Corpse Pose – Five to twenty minutes.

FAT-BURNING SEQUENCE

This includes poses that massage and tone the organs and glands that contribute to better endocrine function, so I am including them in the ultimate fat-burning sequence. You do not need to do all of these poses every session. But since they are all so effective at helping you achieve your weight loss goal, every pose should be done at least twice a week.

POSE	Name and amount of time you should stay in pose
	Child's Pose – One to two minutes, center yourself and breathe.
	Cat–Cow Stretch – Ten times – Arch and flex, with breathing.
	Sun Salutations – Three or four rounds to get warmed up. Be sure to "marry" each movement with either an inhale or an exhale.
	Downward Facing Dog Pose – One minute.
	Bow Pose – Thirty seconds.

	Bridge Pose – Three to five breaths.
	Chair Pose – Three to five breaths.
	Crescent Pose – Three to five breaths, each side.
	Twisting Crescent Lunge Pose – Three to five breaths, each side.
	Thigh Stretch – Three to five breaths, each side.
	Lord of the Dance Pose – Three to five breaths, each side.
	Warrior III – Three to five breaths.
	Plank Pose – Three to five breaths, each side.

	Upward Plank – Three to five breaths.
	Seated Twist Pose – Five to ten breaths, each side.
	Boat Pose – Three to five breaths.
	Plow Pose – Five breaths.
	Shoulder Stand – One to three minutes.
	Happy Baby Pose – One minute.
	Corpse Pose – Five to twenty minutes.

Chapter 8

The Easy Weight Loss Yoga Style of Eating

Keep in mind that in order to lose weight, all systems must be working optimally, or at least successfully, for you to be getting the most nutrients from your food. Only then will you be able to have adequate energy to move through your day and ample enough to practice yoga. To be able to achieve "effortless" weight loss, your goal should be to constantly have nutrients slowly being released into your blood stream. For that, you must eat regularly and eat the right foods. Fortunately, the foods that enable the slow drip of nutrients into your system are also the ones that can help you shed pounds. And if you continue to eat them for the rest of your life, you'll naturally shed your excess weight and stay slim and healthy.

In addition, practicing yoga will contribute to the desire to eat lighter, healthier foods, and you might even want to explore vegetarianism, which is the dietary discipline that most serious yogis adhere to. The digestion and assimilation of meat is more difficult and takes more energy than that of vegetables and dairy products. It can be an interesting experiment for you to challenge your assumptions and beliefs about what kinds of food you need to eat for health, strength, and happiness, and it will give you insights into yourself as you progress with your yoga program.

EAT THE RIGHT FOODS TO BURN OFF YOUR EXCESS FAT STORES

Here's something to ponder—if you put diesel or aviation fuel in a gas-burning car, how long would it run at optimal efficiency? It might get you a few miles before sputtering and giving out, because the car is not meant to run on that type of fuel. By the same token, your body evolved to eat certain kinds of foods, and it will run for years on low-grade "fuel," but unless you give it the kinds of maximum-efficiency foods it needs, it will not operate at its best and will accumulate all kinds of toxic byproducts that will lessen your quality of life. Your body will use any kind of crappy fuel you give it and do the best it can, for a certain period of time. Remember when you were a teenager, when you could eat all the junk you wanted, never gain an ounce, and had boundless energy? However, now that you're in your thirties, forties, fifties, or beyond, the stubborn additional poundage refuses to budge and the buildup of toxins and fat are like sludge in a lean, serene machine, draining your "go" power.

From an evolutionary standpoint, your body is meant to burn two types of fuel—sugar or fat, and it actually runs best on fat instead of sugar. Although either fuel works, fat is the best energy source, releasing more than twice as much energy than is released by burning sugar, because it releases far fewer damaging elements called "free radicals" than does burning sugar/carbohydrates for the same amount of energy. So fat is the fuel we should primarily be utilizing. You want to coax your body into utilizing your excess fat as energy, then continue to use the fat you consume in food as your primary energy source for the rest of your life.

To make this point very clear, here are some additional comparison points regarding burning fat versus sugar:

SUGAR

- Lesser amount of energy is produced for the amount of material burned.

- Burns very fast and produces a lot of wasted energy in the form of damaging free radicals.

Our cells were designed to burn sugar only temporarily in times of emergency, when the damage from free radicals is not as important as dealing with the situation (like a wooly mammoth chasing you).

If our bodies had been designed to primarily burn sugar as a fuel, then we would store sugar cubes within our bodies, but we don't. We store fat. We store only minor amounts of sugar (in our muscles, in the form of glycogen)—enough to last for thirty to sixty minutes of exertion.

When we are asleep, there is no incoming sugar, so those people whose bodies are in a sugar-burning mode dismantle bone and muscle to obtain sugar to burn for energy during sleep. This causes muscle and bone loss, and is a primary factor in osteoporosis.

Being in a sugar-burning mode causes an elevation of sugar in the blood, which causes an alteration of proteins (glycation) and damage to our tissues.

FAT

- Greater energy is produced for the amount of material burned.

- The amount of free radicals released as byproducts of energy creation is less.

- Bone and muscle integrity is maintained because fat is being burned for energy.

- Fat can come directly from food eaten, or the body can get fat from our stored fat (which is exactly what we want for fat loss).

This is very important, because we need energy even if we haven't been able to eat in the last few hours, such as when we are asleep.

Unfortunately, most people's cells have been "conditioned" to burn sugar, with a whole host of resulting negative consequences. The bodies of sugar-burning people (you are a sugar burner if you have a lot of abdominal fat and cravings for sugar) often have large amounts of stored fat, but the cells of their bodies ignore that fat and look only for sugar. If there is no sugar available, such as when you're sleeping, then the body will dismantle bones and muscles and convert those proteins in sugar to be burned for energy. As I mentioned, this is one of the major causes of muscle loss and osteoporosis as we get older.

The unhealthy situation of being a sugar burner results because the hypothalamus (the energy-controlling gland in the brain) signals the cells of our bodies to only burn sugar instead of fat—the result of leptin hormone levels that have gone so high that the hypothalamus becomes unable to understand the leptin signals. (Remember that leptin is a messenger molecule made in fat cells, which communicates to the hypothalamus to inform how much energy is stored in the body). Controlling leptin levels is the key to body fat management.

When leptin levels are high, the cells of the body become both leptin and insulin resistant. You will find it difficult to keep your blood sugar at normal levels, begin to age much more quickly, have extra fat that you cannot lose, and be susceptible to diseases such as diabetes. Diabetes is a metabolic disease in which the body's inability to produce any or enough insulin causes elevated levels of glucose in the blood. Elevated levels of glucose in the blood then causes hyperglycemia, which, when occurring frequently or for long periods of time, causes damage to nerves, blood vessels, and other body organs.

Unless leptin levels are conditioned to stay at a lower level, you will find that you continue gaining fat over the years until your fat cells become resistant to leptin and insulin. When your cells are no longer able to handle excess glucose in the blood, you set the stage for possible diabetes and all its attendant health issues.

CHANGING INTO A LEAN, SERENE, FAT BURNING MACHINE

How to Go From Sugar Burning to Fat Burning

One of the wisest health habits you can adopt is to eat in a way that lowers your leptin levels and repairs the damage done to the hypothalamus, so that it will instruct the cells of your body to burn fat instead of sugar. In the simplest terms, the way to do this is:

- Eat very little sugar
- Limit amounts of starchy carbohydrates, including bread, pasta, rice, and potatoes
- Eat generous amounts of good fats, such as olive, coconut, and red palm oil
- Eat sufficient amounts of protein
- Eat high amounts of non-starchy vegetables

For most people, training the hypothalamus to be sensitive to leptin again is a matter of retraining oneself to eat a better way.[15]

If you are presently a sugar burner and want to become a fat burner, you must avoid sugar/simple carbohydrates completely for at least a month. At the same time, you must reduce your leptin levels by other means (via exercise, diet, and stress reduction) until your hypothalamus is able to put your cells back into the fat-burning mode.

You can learn more about the "low" or "slow" carb style of eating by exploring something called the "Primal Eating" or the "Paleo Diet" concept, which is gaining quite a foothold in the health and wellness community and involves eating the way our ancestors ate. No, that doesn't mean we have to rip away at raw meat or cook over an open flame, but it does suggest we should eat in the same way that allowed our fore-bears to evolve. That means we must pay attention to limiting our body's insulin response. Our ancestors did this without realizing they were doing it.

Research puts our primal ancestors' carb count at about 80 grams per day, compared to the average American's 350 to 500 grams per day. The low-carb, low-sugar diet resulted in the body creating several ways to make extra insulin but only one way to get rid of it. Thus, when we pack in the carbs today, based on popular high-carb foods are the biggest culprits—cereal products, high-fructose corn syrup, processed

---

15 *http://www.healthy-living.org/html/be_a_fat_burner.html*

foods, and fast food staples such as hamburgers and French fries—we are creating a lot of extra insulin that builds up in our blood and bodies, initially stored as sugar but soon stored as fat. Our blood sugar levels tend to go haywire when we keep piling in the carbs and sugar. Primal eating instead focuses on keeping the blood sugar level even, with a slow trickle of nutrients into the bloodstream over the course of the day, preventing the spikes and valleys in your blood sugar levels, as well as controlling insulin overload.

If you want to find out more, two excellent resources on the subject are Timothy Ferriss' *The Four Hour Body*, and *The Primal Blueprint* by Mark Sisson.

YOU NEED TO EAT FAT TO LOSE FAT

Your body has a choice of fuels depending on the situation. In an emergency, or if the body needs energy fast, it chooses sugar as its fuel. Sugar is stored mostly in the muscles and the blood stream so it's readily available. During any prolonged physical activity, the body always burns sugar for approximately the first twelve minutes. At that twelve-minute mark, the body then decides whether to keep burning sugar or to switch fuels and to start burning fat.

Eating less fat means you must eat more protein or carbs, and most people end up eating more carbs (and the wrong type). Dietary fat is very slow burning in the body so when you replace the fat with faster-burning carbs, you tend to feel less energetic, risk burning muscle tissue, and wreak havoc on your metabolism and hormones because your energy levels (blood sugar) are like a roller coaster.

Dietary fats supply some of the best and most stable sources of energy. So if you want to feel good all day long, you need to make sure you are getting enough fats, and the right types. The best types of fat include:

Fish – Fish like salmon, albacore tuna, herring, mackerel, and sardines, which contain beneficial amounts of omega-3 fatty acids.

Oils – Heart-healthy oils like cod liver, olive, canola, and peanut oil are excellent sources of fat for dieters. They have also been shown to lower bad cholesterol and reduce the risk of heart disease. Use oils sparingly when sautéing or for salads. Moderation is important. You really only need about a teaspoon of oil to get the benefits. Using more will add significant calories, and portion control is still important.

Avocados – Add avocado to a spinach and carrot salad, and you'll not only get a dose of good fat, but you'll also absorb more phytonutrients like lutein and beta-carotene. Scientists at Ohio State University in Columbus found that more antioxidants were absorbed when people ate a salad containing avocados than when they ate a salad without it. One quarter of an avocado will add flavor while only adding about seventy-five calories. Many people are unaware that avocados are also high in fiber.

Nuts – Almonds, walnuts, pecans, and peanuts are powerhouses of good nutrition—full of antioxidants, minerals, and monounsaturated fat. The Nurses Health Study, where more than 86,000 nurses were followed for fourteen years, found that those who ate nuts regularly (about an ounce per day) tended to weigh less than those who didn't. The protein, fat, and fiber make nuts more filling, which helps dieters stay on track. Plus there's a psychological bonus to eating nuts—they're rich and satisfying, and most people associate them with parties.

Flaxseeds – Packing the triple wallop of beneficial fat, protein, and fiber, flaxseeds are a delicious and healthful addition to any diet. You can grind them up and add them to oatmeal, yogurt, salads, or vegetables, or pretty much anywhere you want a nutty crunch. They're a plant source of omega-3 fatty acids, making them a good choice for vegetarians or non-fish-loving folks. Ground flaxseeds also have three grams of fiber per tablespoon, which helps slow digestion and keep your blood sugar stable.[16]

The human body needs fat just to function properly, let alone to achieve optimal health. As we've seen above, certain amounts of fat are necessary for proper hormone production. If hormone production is off,

---

16 *Melody Garza MS RD CISSN, http://sportsnutritioninsider.insidefit-nessmag.com/3855/the-fab-five-fats-for-getting-lean*

your metabolism will be off too. Hormones regulate many things in the body, including your ability to build and maintain muscle tissue, which is responsible for a large portion of your energy expenditure. In simple terms, muscle burns calories twenty-four hours a day, and if you eat a low-fat or no-fat diet you will have a hard time building and maintaining muscle.

HOW TO TRAIN YOUR BODY TO BURN FAT, NOT SUGAR

How does your body make the decision to switch fuels? It's a function of your activity level, and your body uses your heart rate to make the decision. If you are working or exercising at an aerobic level, the body will always choose to burn sugar. If you are working or exercising at a slower, sub-aerobic level, your body can take it easy and make the switch to burning fat. The trick is that fat burns more slowly than sugar.

So you can see what happens. If you're doing high-energy aerobics (high heart rate), you will only burn sugar. This explains why people can do a lot of aerobics and still have an unhealthy high percentage of body fat. When you do aerobic exercise at a high heart rate, you are only burning sugar for energy, not fat.

The ideal heart rate for burning fat can be generated by practicing yoga at about 70 percent, between your top aerobic zone and your maximum heart rate. If you're in your thirties or forties, that's about

130 (about 120 if you're older), which is very easy to reach doing yoga at a moderate pace. For example, if you are forty years old, your maximum heart rate would be approximately 180 beats per minute, and your aerobic heart rate at 85 percent would be 153. So if you were to work at a moderate 70 percent of your maximum heart rate, your target heart rate during your yoga practice would be 126 beats per minute.

The chart below shows the aerobic level and the resting level for your age that can help you determine your ideal heart rate for optimum fat burning.[17]

Target Heart Rate Maximum Target Training Zones							
	Approximate maximum heart rate	Maximum target training zones (beats per minute)					
Age	Heart rate	60%	65%	70%	75%	80%	85%
20	200	120	130	140	150	160	170
25	195	117	127	137	146	156	166
30	190	114	124	133	143	152	162
35	185	111	120	130	139	148	157
40	180	108	117	126	135	144	153
45	175	105	114	123	131	140	149
50	170	102	111	119	128	136	145
55	165	99	107	116	124	132	140
60	160	96	104	112	120	128	136
65	155	93	101	109	116	124	132
70	150	90	98	105	113	120	128
75	145	87	94	102	109	116	123
80	140	84	91	98	105	112	119

17 Source: *Allina Patient Education, Basic Skills for Living with Diabetes,* fifth edition, ISBN 1-931876-32-0

CHAPTER 9

Breathing, Meditation, and Focusing Techniques

Although the physical poses may be the most well-known element of Hatha Yoga, yoga masters will tell you they're not the entire point of yoga practice. According to yoga philosophy, the postures exist to open the body for more energy to flow through it and aid in introducing us to deeper states of meditation that lead toward enlightenment, where our minds can grow perfectly still and our lives become content. But just how do we make the leap from Downward Dog to divine bliss? Ancient texts give us a clear answer: breathe like a yogi. It has been said that yoga practice is more correctly "breathing with postures," rather than postures with breathing.

Our breathing can mirror our psychological state in any given moment. If you don't think you need help in this area, spot check your normal breathing pattern at various points throughout the day. Notice how you breathe while you're driving, sitting at your desk, walking down the block, or fighting with your spouse. Unless you've been practicing pranayama, chances are you have one or more unconscious negative breathing habits.

THE MOST COMMON BAD BREATHING HABITS AND HOW TO CORRECT THEM

Improper breathing habits can leave you with low levels of energy, high levels of irritability, a weak immune system, and loads of stress. Shallow breathing and upper-chest breathing are two of the more common bad breathing habits. Neither allows you to use the full power or capacity of your breath. If your inhalations and exhalations do not move your lower ribs one iota, you're practicing the former. If only your chest moves when you breathe, leaving your abdomen immobile, you're guilty of the latter.

The worst of the bad breathing habits is breath holding, which consists of either not breathing at all or holding an inhalation for an extended period of time—both of which tending to happen when we are fearful or stressed. When this occurs, you cut yourself off from the most life-sustaining substance known to humanity—oxygen.

Short and choppy breathing can also deprive your body of its most important element, and in most situations, this kind of breath results in a frustrating experience. Over-breathing (hyperventilation) is breathing too much, which upsets the balance of gases in your system and happens when you take in too much oxygen and do not expel enough carbon dioxide. Exhalations should take a slightly longer length of time than the inhalations and be completely relaxed, in order to provoke the relaxation response. Most of us, however, most likely engage in under-breathing for various reasons.

The bad habit of mouth breathing occurs when you totally ignore your nasal passage and only inhale and exhale from your mouth.

Reverse breathing, as the name implies, actually reverses the natural movement of your diaphragm and abdomen. An exhalation should leave your abdomen slightly flattened, while an inhalation should slightly raise it. Reverse breathing does the opposite. Watch a baby breathe. Its shoulders don't go up and down; its little tummy goes in and out.

BREATHING AWARENESS

In building a foundation to establish the basics of breathing, you must first understand that they are not so much breathing *techniques* as they are methods of establishing basic breath *awareness* and elimination of bad habits and irregularities. Breath awareness is so important that, in a sense, you can say that the whole science of breath begins and ends with mindful awareness.

Bad breathing habits tend to crop up during times of stress, like when you're in an intense discussion or have had an auto accident. These include holding the breath; jerky, ragged breathing; short and choppy exhalations; and tensing the muscles in the upper chest, shoulders, and throat, constricting the breath and literally leave us gasping for air. You can get rid of the stress by learning to literally breathe easy. Think of your breathing rhythm as a lullaby that gently lulls your mind into a state of calm.

PROGRESSIVE RELAXATION BREATHING TECHNIQUE

Here's a simple way to calm your body and keep it quiet during stressful times:

Spend about a minute and, in your mind, scan through your body with your inner awareness to notice any areas of tension or holding.

Go through a step-by-step conscious relaxation process, starting with intentionally relaxing your jaw, followed by your throat, neck, shoulders, arms, belly, spine, hips and legs.

Inhale deeply, and imagine the breath reaching to the deepest part of your torso, all the way down to where your lungs end, slightly above your waist.

Exhale deeply and relax. Focus on letting go of any area in which you have noticed tension.

Repeat ten times, scanning your interior landscape for any area that you're holding on to, and breathe toward that spot.

Breath awareness builds the bridge between the

body and the mind. When trying to still the mind, it is extremely common to notice muscular tension and exceptionally noisy thoughts. The busy thoughts are actually there all the time, but it is not until you focus on and attempt to quiet your mind that you notice how clamoring they really are.

The nervous system is what controls the interface. One of the best ways to regulate your nervous system, and in turn the body and mind, is through the breath. This has been known by yogis for thousands of years, and has also come to be widely known in recent years by the modern medical and psychological community, and now by you.

COUNTING BREATHS PRANAYAMA EXERCISE

An ideal way to practice both efficient breathing habits and calming the mind is with a pranayama exercise where you breathe in, out, and hold the breath for specific counts.

- Close your eyes and breathe using the following count:
- Inhale deeply for four counts;
- hold for four counts;
- exhale fully for six counts; and
- hold without breathing for two counts.

(Note: If you have high blood pressure or any kind

of heart problem, do not hold your breath; just make the inhale and exhale eight counts each.)

Allow each muscle in your body to relax, consciously focus on letting go, unwinding, and releasing any tension. Use the progressive muscle breathing technique we described above to bring down your tension level a few notches.

Practice this for five to ten minutes, and notice what a difference it makes. If you find that you get agitated during your counting pranayama breathing exercise, it could possibly be because you are breathing too fast or forcing the exhale out too hard. If this happens, just make the breathing gentler.

EXERCISE FOR FOCUS AND CONCENTRATION

Find a quiet place where you can sit comfortably and you won't be disturbed for at least five to ten minutes. Shut off your cell phone, close the door, and do your best to otherwise eliminate any potential distractions or interruptions. Find an object to hold—it can be anything, a small statue, a rock, a flower, or even a nail clipper. (Avoid an object with words on it, like a magazine, which you will be tempted to read.) Close your eyes and practice the Counting Pranayama exercise you just learned for about three minutes.

Then open your eyes and place your awareness on the object in your hand. Gaze at it. Examine it deeply, noticing the color, texture, weight, and any specific details. Note the size of the object, the depth, the pattern, any scratches or mars, or other interesting qualities. Continue to examine the object deeply for a few minutes. If you are aware of any self-induced judging or comparing, just breathe and bring your awareness back to the object. If your mind starts to wander, just notice it when it does and, without criticizing yourself, gently bring your concentration back to the object.

Now close your eyes and imagine the object as you just examined it. Try to recall every aspect you noted with your eyes open. If you notice you're having thoughts, open your eyes again, place your attention and awareness on the object, then close your eyes again, and continue recalling the details. After three minutes of this focus and concentration exercise, open your eyes and notice how you feel. You will probably feel clearer and refreshed.

BECOMING MORE MINDFUL

What Does "Mindfulness" Mean?

Mindfulness is our ability to be aware of what is going on both inside us and around us. It is the continuous awareness of our bodies, emotions, and thoughts.

In the Sutra on the Four Establishments of Mindfulness, the Buddha offers four layers of mindfulness practice: mindfulness of the body, of the emotions, of the mind, and of the objects of mind.

Practicing mindfulness at each layer can be the foundation of well-being and happiness.

When we don't practice mindfulness, we suffer in our body, our mind, and in our relationships. In practicing mindfulness, we become a peaceful refuge for ourselves and others. When the seed of mindfulness in us is watered, it can grow into enlightenment, understanding, compassion, and transformation. The more we practice mindfulness, the stronger this seed will grow.

Clarity flows from mindfulness. With the energy of mindfulness, we can always return to our true home, the present moment. Mindfulness helps us to come back to the here and now, to be aware of what is going on in the present moment, and to be in touch with the wonders of life.[18]

Focusing on one task at a time, putting yourself fully into that task, is much more effective than multitasking. Focusing on one task at a time is also more satisfying. I've proven it to myself time and again over the last few years. Focusing on what you're doing right now is more effective than when you are switching back and forth between several conversations or tasks. You become more productive when you're mindful.

But more importantly, being present is undoubtedly the only way to enjoy life to the fullest. By being present, you enjoy your food more, you enjoy friends

18 *An excerpt from Mindful Movements: Ten Exercises For Well-Being by Thich Nhat Hanh, Gaiam Life website, life.gaiam.com*

and family more, you enjoy anything you're doing more. Even things you might think are drudgery or boring, such as housework, can be amazing if you are truly present. Try it—wash dishes or sweep or cook and remain fully present. It takes practice, but it's incredible.[19]

_____

19 Leo Babauta, April 29, 2009, *http://zenhabits.net/*

CONCLUSION

To manifest the changes that you want in your life, you must be motivated enough to consistently do things differently than you have in the past. If indeed, you are not willing to get yourself onto the mat for at least thirty minutes, four to five times a week, preferring instead to watch TV or another pursuit, then your results will be insignificant and life will go on much as it has in the past.

Please don't tell yourself that you want to start a program and then allow it to lamely peter out due to lack of motivation; it will just make you feel worse than ever. Remember my saying that SIBTN (Something is Better than Nothing) and try to bring to mind the sense of accomplishment and well-being that you'll get when you've completed your yoga session. Let that feeling draw you along the path of health and quality of life.

Happily, allowing yourself to become immersed in the discipline of yoga, no matter how deeply you immerse yourself, will transform your body and draw you seductively along a path of inner peace and evolution of your being. It will give you more than a slimmer body—it will give you a refreshed outlook and new zest for life. The changing of focus from all that exists outside of "you," to the inner landscape, the eternal "Beingness," gives you inner peace and renewed enthusiasm to tackle the challenges of life. It will begin to happen spontaneously when you make the initial effort. When you take the time to connect with the Life Force energy within, your efforts will be rewarded with ever-greater inner peace, wellness, creativity, and expression.

When you spend time "on the mat" daily, you will be sensitive to yourself and others, more compassionate, and more willing to make changes for the better. As you connect daily with the Force of which you are a part, your wisdom grows and you begin to see your daily challenges in a new light, with renewed respect for the challenges that you have overcome.

You will begin to feel inwardly strong, and the original quest that started your yoga course—the desire to get thinner—will begin to fall away as you are carried along a path by a larger quest, that of the desire to know yourself and your purpose.

The idea of knowing yourself and your purpose should be uppermost, knowing who you are and why you're here on Earth, at this time, in this body, with your particular mind, strengths, and experiences. You will get to know your inner landscape and be able to "tend to" your inner garden, making changes as needed for your own well-being and happiness.

You cannot practice yoga without your life changing. The idea of "practice" falls away, and yoga just becomes part of your life, a part so closely intertwined with who you are that you will wonder how you ever lived without it. If you let it, yoga can make your life better in so many ways. Why? Don't ask me. Yoga just does that.

To My Readers

Before you go, I'd like to say thank you for purchasing and reading my book. I know that you have a choice among dozens of books on Amazon, but you took a chance with mine, and I hope you enjoyed it. So here's a big thank-you for downloading this ebook or audiobook and getting all the way to the end.

Now I'd like to ask you for a small favor. If you loved or even just liked the print, e- or audiobook, could you please take a minute or two and leave a review or your comments? Your feedback will help others who want to make positive changes in their life, who may be struggling with overweight, negative body image, or compulsive overeating/bingeing disorders. Your review or positive comments will also help me to continue in creating the kind of books and media that will help you get results.

Thank you again. You can reach me anytime with questions or comments at pb@vivationusa.com or toll-free at 800-931-7007.

Additional Books and Media from Benesserra Publishing

The New Weight Loss Blueprint

You CAN lose weight and keep it off, but not by dieting...by firing up your hormonal system! Learn how you can lose weight effortlessly with the fifteen power foods your body craves. Diets don't work! The last thing you want to do is put on MORE fat by actually eliminating the systems that will enable you to burn your excess fat for energy. That's what you do when you starve yourself on a restricted-calorie diet—or worse, go on a diet that has you eating only grapefruit for a week.

Your body will stubbornly insist on holding on to its fat stores. To be successful at weight loss, you must gently coax the pounds off by making a few simple and easy changes. Weight loss is easy when your metabolic system is working correctly. That's why you need to be "healthy" before you can be "slim."

So, it's not a dramatic, but slow continual weight loss, where you can effortlessly lose twelve pounds a year. Pretty thrilling!

Vivation Supercharge Your Life CD Set

Vivation is the emotional skill of harmonizing your emotions to create happiness and peace of mind. Learning Vivation can make an enormous, lasting difference in the quality of your life. Using your breath and skills that you already have, you can resolve long-held negative emotions on your own with this wonderful and refreshing technique. Unlike anything you've ever tried, Vivation supercharges your life, giving you a tool that can be used anytime to feel better about yourself, optimistic, and enthusiastic about life.

Vivation for Prosperity Volumes 1 and 2

Change your relationship to money! In just a few hours, you can radically shift the limiting factors that prevent you from creating the prosperity you desire. Vivation is a powerful breathwork and awareness technique for healing your negative emotions about abundance. Doing Vivation will increase your income, happiness, effectiveness, creativity, and peace of mind. Vivation allows you to relax deeply, have better health and relationships, permanently increase your self-esteem, and go after and get more of whatever you want in life. You'll feel so good about yourself, nothing will stop you!

Vivation for Prosperity Volume 1 is an explanation of the breathwork process, to prepare you to begin healing your relationship to money. You need both volumes to learn and do Vivation for Prosperity.

In the first volume, Patricia explains the Five Elements of Vivation. You will learn what causes negativity, how your relationship to your feelings affects your prosperity, and how the Five Elements of

Vivation enable you to intentionally create emotional resolution of your troubling emotions. By discovering the source of your "lack," you are able to overcome the reasons you keep yourself poor.

The second CD is a guided session of Vivation breathwork. As you continue to use it, Vivation will support you in permanently changing your consciousness about abundance and money.

Food Addicts

Do you eat for emotional reasons? Do you "use" food as a barrier to feelings? Have you all but given up on ever achieving your ideal body? The top ten tips in Food Addicts will show you how to end compulsive eating, lose weight, keep it off, and give you the confidence you need to take charge of your life!

You'll learn why dieting never works in the long run for weight loss, how emotions masquerade as hunger and how to tell the difference between the two, how to eliminate fear and anxiety about food and eating; and how to reach your ideal weight without dieting or deprivation!

You don't need another diet...you need emotional rescue to resolve the underlying reasons you overeat.

You can stop "using" food to solve problems it can't solve and start feeling good when you see results, without the need for self-restriction and denial. If you're sick of the depressing downward spiral that dieting creates and are ready to heal the underlying causes of your out-of-control eating, you owe it to yourself to try this powerful solution that will not only be the end of dieting forever, but make you a happier, stronger person with high self-esteem. Then you can go after and get what you really need to satisfy your hunger for living!

Easy Weight Loss Yoga 1

Find out how the ancient practice of yoga can help you get swimsuit sexy by stepping up your metabolism, adding muscle, and eliminating toxins and unwanted fat. Learn the poses that will shed pounds while toning up the organs and glands that make you a lean, serene, fat-burning machine. You'll relax better and become focused, strong, and energized. Diets alone never work for lasting weight loss, and repeated dieting causes metabolic and psychological damage. Let's face it, no one likes to diet; you simply need to outsmart your metabolism to lose weight and keep it off. Find out the secrets of how to coax your body into using up its fat stores for energy, not saving them as extra flab on your hips. Includes motivational tips to keep you "on the mat" and explains how important proper breathing is to achieving the healthy, lithe, and sexy body you've always wanted. Get started now to be bikini-ready in a few short months. No yoga experience necessary—you can dive in at any level with these twelve easy poses. Illustrated.

Play Better Golf with Easy Yoga

Powerful, proven, and effective—discover the path to par with easy yoga!

- Improve balance and body positioning.

- Increase swing distance and accuracy.

- Gain stamina and energy.

- Calm the overactive, "critical" mind.

- Avoid golf-related injuries to joints and spine.

- Enjoy the game more...even from the rough!

Golf pros everywhere are using and recommending yoga to provide a comprehensive workout, aid in mastering the mental game, and foster more consistent play. On and off the course, golfers who practice yoga enjoy greater confidence, power, and focus.

Learn special breathing techniques to calm the mind and relax the body, leading to tireless, effortless play and greater shot distance and control.

Strengthen your core and enhance muscle memory and increase flexibility, reducing the risk of golf-related injury and shortening recovery time.

Illustrated, easy-to-follow, yoga-based fitness exercises help you find—and stay in—your zone. Lower your score and your blood pressure...the easy way.

Loving Yourself Thin

Do you feel out of control—a compulsive eater with a negative body image or low self-esteem? Diets don't work; they never do! It's time to eliminate the causes of overeating, overweight, and fat, and lose the weight once and forever.

Learn how to achieve your ideal body without dieting or deprivation. This organic, no-diet method makes you lose your desire to ever overeat. This large-format workbook provides an easy and comprehensive ten-week plan for healing underlying negative emotions and losing weight effortlessly. Simply read one chapter a week, do the exercises at the end of each chapter, and transform yourself into a more confident, slimmer person. When you stop using food to solve problems in your life, the excess weight will simply begin to fall away!

Loving Yourself Thin with Vivation Breathwork CD Set

Experience the powerful and profound effect of Vivation breathwork—your personal emotional healing turbocharger—and start feeling good about yourself. You'll be able to finally lose weight, keep it off, and get more of what you really crave in life.

With this CD set and the Loving Yourself Thin ten-week workbook, you'll have everything you need to start your last-ever weight loss program and the beginning of a happier life. The long-awaited audio companion to Patricia Bacall's Loving Yourself Thin workbook, the Loving Yourself Thin with Vivation Breathwork CD set gives you the tools you need to stop using food to solve life's problems, feel good about yourself, lose weight, and keep it off.

With disc 1, you will hear Patricia, an internationally recognized authority on emotional healing and a world-renowned wellness expert, explain the powerful, life-changing Vivation technique. With disc 2, she will guide you through a complete Vivation breathwork session. In just minutes, you will feel more relaxed and positive. By the end of the session, you will have profound breakthroughs that enable you to love yourself more at any size and finally end your struggle with dieting, overeating, and negative body image. You will radically change your relationship to food and eating, gently begin to let go of the excess weight that you've been holding on to, put a stop to dieting, and live at your ideal weight forever.

The Chocolate Lovers Guide to Weight Loss

A fun and seriously effective way to end dieting. Reach your ideal weight without effort and struggle, including dozens of tips and shortcuts to enhance your metabolism, burn more calories, build muscle, and work out more effectively. Learn how you can eat real food and enjoy life while eating the foods you love, including chocolate!

Vivation – The Skill of Happiness

Kindle ebook by Jim Leonard

Vivation IS the skill of happiness. It brings together the breath and focused awareness to empower you on many levels. Vivation enables you to experience a superior life by removing negative factors from your subconscious mind. Specifically, Vivation causes integration—the ability to happily accept reality while empowering you to change the situation if desired.

Thousands worldwide are using this wonderful and powerful process invented by Jim Leonard, who personally facilitated more than forty-thousand Vivation sessions in twenty countries in his lifetime. This is his third and most definitive book on the subject of Vivation.

Acknowledgements

I wish to thank the individuals who helped me with this book, including:

My dedicated and steadfast photographer, Michael Garver

My stalwart yoga models, Lisa Thompson, Don Dawson, and Bruno Lacombe

My eagle-eyed editor, Christy Distler

My meditation teacher, Kathie Jordan, and her husband Jim Jordan

I wish to also extend my heartfelt gratitude to the dedicated and wonderful yoga teachers with whom I have practiced and learned.

About Patricia Bacall

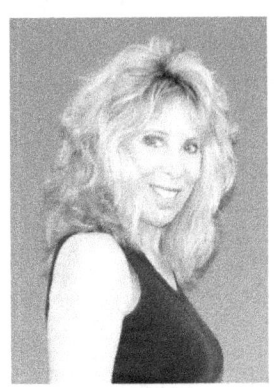

Patricia Bacall is an internationally acknowledged authority in the field of personal growth, and teaches individuals and group classes throughout the world on how to live happier, more fulfilling and creative lives, attracting people of all backgrounds and ages.

As a personal coach and workshop leader, Patricia has a practical approach that is both engaging and intuitive. She is known for her ability to resonate with people and empower them to live freer and more satisfying lives. Participants often comment on her clarity of communication and thorough knowledge of her subject matter.

With her gentle and positive approach, she assists in healing by teaching people to love and appreciate themselves as strong and unique individuals, and to use that self-love as the means to achieve their dreams and goals.

Patricia's journey began in 1980 as a personal trainer, educating individuals to improve their fitness, health and wellbeing. Realizing the importance of the mind-body connection and the healing benefits of yoga, she became a certified yoga instructor and massage therapist.

During the late '80s, Patricia learned the Vivation

breathwork technique, which helps people create resolution of their most negative emotions using a simple yet exceptionally powerful process. Working extensively with Jim Leonard, the founder of Vivation®, she became one of the best-trained breathwork professionals in the United States. Patricia uses the Vivation technique in her workshops and practice to "supercharge" the healing process by uncovering and resolving suppressed emotions.

To round out her education in body, mind and spirit wellness, Patricia has extensively studied yoga, Pilates, massage, and EFT, and holds several credentials in these disciplines. She serves on the board of the Associated Vivation Professionals in the United States and is a contributor to personal health publications and websites on the subjects of emotional overeating, physical vitality, overcoming emotional negativity, energy work and yoga.

www.ingramcontent.com/pod-product-compliance
Lightning Source LLC
Chambersburg PA
CBHW070416290526
45791CB00005B/1724